YOUNG WOMEN WITH ADHD

SIMPLE STEPS TO IDENTIFY TRAITS, KEEP IMPULSES IN CHECK, EMBRACE NEURODIVERSITY & DEVELOP EXECUTIVE FUNCTIONING SKILLS

RO SIRISENA

Copyright © 2023. All rights reserved.

The content within this book may not be reproduced, duplicated, or transmitted without direct written permission from the author or the publisher.

Under no circumstances will any blame or legal responsibility be held against the publisher, or author, for any damages, reparation, or monetary loss due to the information contained within this book, either directly or indirectly.

Legal Notice:

This book is copyright protected. It is only for personal use. You cannot amend, distribute, sell, use, quote, or paraphrase any part of the content within this book, without the consent of the author or publisher.

Disclaimer Notice:

Please note the information contained within this document is for educational and entertainment purposes only. All effort has been expended to present accurate, up-to-date, reliable, and complete information. No warranties of any kind are declared or implied. Readers acknowledge that the author is not engaged in the rendering of legal, financial, medical, or professional advice. The content within this book has been derived from various sources. Please consult a licensed professional before attempting any techniques outlined in this book.

By reading this document, the reader agrees that under no circumstances is the author responsible for any losses, direct or indirect, that are incurred as a result of the use of the information contained within this document, including, but not limited to, errors, omissions, or inaccuracies.

CONTENTS

1. UNDERSTANDING ADHD — 7
   - Ava — 7
   - Debunking Myths — 8
   - So, What Is ADHD? — 11
   - Causes Of ADHD — 12
   - The Neuroscience Of The ADHD Brain — 14
   - The ADHD Brain vs. A Neurotypical Brain — 15
   - Symptoms, Diagnosis, And Treatment — 17
   - It's Different For Women — 24
   - What ADHD Looks Like In Women — 27
   - Mental Health Conditions That Commonly Occur With ADHD In Adult Women — 29
   - Summary — 31

2. ADHD IS NOT SO BAD — 33
   - It's Not So Bad Afterall - Inside Ava's Head — 33
   - Things to Love About Your ADHD — 35
   - Women With ADHD Who Rock — 41
   - You Are Not The Sum Of It All — 44
   - How To Regain Your Confidence — 50
   - Summary — 53

3. HEALTH & SELF-CARE — 55
   - The Week I've Had! — 55
   - Your Lifestyle Will Determine Your Future — 56
   - Get Enough Sleep — 56
   - Healthy Eating — 62
   - Physical Exercise — 71
   - Stress Management — 75
   - Mindfulness and ADHD — 90
   - Summary — 93

4. MANAGING EMOTIONS & REJECTION SENSITIVITY — 95

A Decade Lost	95
Exaggerated Emotions	96
Emotional Regulation And Redirection	100
Rejection Sensitivity	104
What About Empathy?	107
The Power Of Gratitude	114
Summary	122

5. IMPROVING YOUR RELATIONSHIP WITH MONEY

	123
It's Harder to Manage Finances	124
Financial Management	127
Saving And Spending	133
Avoid Impulsive Spending	137
Summary	141

6. A MORE LIVABLE HOME

	143
Clitter-Clutter	143
ADHD And Messiness	144
Decluttering	145
ADHD-Friendly Ways Of Getting Organized	148
Summary	155

7. ADHD AT WORK

	157
Upside-Down Ethic	157
Symptoms Posing Problems In the Workplace	158
Should You Let Them Know?	159
Managing Symptoms at Work	163
Time Wasters and Productivity Killers	165
Time Management	169
Summary	174

8. CULTIVATING HEALTHY RELATIONSHIPS & DEVELOPING SOCIAL SKILLS

	175
Love Is An Open Door	175
Mastering Social Skills	176
Social Skills in Adults With ADHD	176
ADHD And Relationships	188
Communication Problems	191

More Relationship Tips: Ways To Save Your Relationship	193
Finding the Right One	195
Summary	198
Conclusion	201
References	205

1

UNDERSTANDING ADHD

AVA

Ava froze. Although she was staring blankly at her computer screen, her brain felt like it was on fire. The email she had just received sent her into a mental frenzy. Suddenly it all seemed too much for her in that moment. At this point, they were all just jumbled letters in her head. Frustrated, she got up from her desk and started to pace. It somehow always made her feel better when she was restless - like now. She glanced back at the computer screen, and with a sigh, she decided to take a break and go for a walk. She would respond to her client later. She couldn't do it right now, even if she tried. She was feeling too frustrated and restless. She always got this way when she started to feel overwhelmed. Ever since she was a sophomore in high school, she had struggled with focusing on one task. Now she was 30 years old, *and nothing had really changed except the frustration that seemed to grow. She had often wondered what was wrong with her, but each time, she would quickly shut down that line of thought. She wasn't ready to confront whatever it was. Maybe someday, soon - she hoped.*

DEBUNKING MYTHS

Like Ava, many women go through their adult lives wondering if there's 'something wrong' with them. And, like Ava, they never really get to the answer. Well, I'm going to help you with some answers. First, I would like to point out that this is in no way, shape, or form meant to be a diagnosis. Whether or not you've been diagnosed with it, ADHD is a condition that can affect anyone, young or adult, male or female. I want to point you in the right direction, make you ask the questions, and take the necessary steps to understand ADHD. I will start with what ADHD is not by debunking some myths.

Myth 1: ADHD is not a real disorder

It's as real as it gets. According to Children and Adults with Attention-Deficit/Hyperactivity Disorder (CHADD), ADHD was identified as far back as 1775. Research using brain scans has shown distinctive variances in brain development between individuals with ADHD and those without the condition. ADHD can hinder essential aspects of daily life, such as social interaction, emotional regulation, academic performance, and job productivity. The condition also has a genetic component, with a 57% chance of a child inheriting ADHD if one of their parents also has it.

Myth 2: ADHD is a disorder of childhood

This couldn't be further from the truth. ADHD persists throughout a person's lifetime, with many individuals experiencing symptoms into adulthood after an initial childhood diagnosis. The condition continues to affect between 50% to 80% of individuals from childhood into adolescence and around 35% to 65% of individuals into adulthood. A study that focused on girls between the ages of 6 and 12 diagnosed with ADHD in childhood discovered that a decade later, these girls still experienced more frequent occurrences of ADHD and additional co-occurring conditions.

Myth 3: ADHD is over-diagnosed

This could be because of the 5% yearly increase in diagnoses, but those diagnosed with ADHD were diagnosed using best practice guidelines. So, the increase in diagnoses could be because of enhanced knowledge and awareness of ADHD among healthcare providers and parents; increased screening efforts by primary care providers; a decline in stigma associated with ADHD; greater availability of effective treatments, and a potential increase in cases related to environmental factors such as exposure to toxins during pregnancy or elevated levels of lead in the blood.

Myth 4: Children with ADHD are over-medicated

Interestingly, it's pretty much the opposite! Medications used to manage ADHD symptoms are considered appropriate and, in other cases, undertreated. A survey of children diagnosed with ADHD showed that only 69% were taking medication to manage symptoms. That's hardly over-medicating, wouldn't you agree?

Myth 5: Poor parenting causes ADHD

Poor parenting has nothing to do with ADHD in children. While parenting practices are not a direct cause of ADHD, they could exacerbate symptoms of co-occurring disorders, such as conduct disorder (CD) and oppositional defiant disorder (ODD). In fact, hereditary and neurological factors, such as pregnancy and birth complications and brain damage, are the real culprits.

Myth 6: Minority Children are over-diagnosed with ADHD and are over-medicated

Contrary to popular belief, white children have the highest rates of ADHD diagnosis based on reports from parents. The prevalence of ADHD diagnosis in white children is 11.5%, compared to 8.9% for black children and 6.3% for Hispanic children. Examining the Early Childhood Longitudinal Study, Kindergarten Class of 1998–1999, revealed that minority children were less prone than white children to receive an ADHD diagnosis. The study also showed that children of Hispanic, African American, or other ethnicities diagnosed with ADHD were significantly less likely to be prescribed medication.

Myth 7: Girls Have Lower Rates and Less Severe ADHD than Boys

It's this one that gets me. It wasn't until recently that ADHD in females has been acknowledged, and more research is now highlighting the significant impairments that they experience, which can be like those of males. Girls are as prone as boys to being diagnosed with ADHD, with a diagnostic rate of 13.3% for boys and 5.6% for girls, according to a survey. Girls with ADHD are vulnerable to many of the same co-occurring conditions and challenges as their male counterparts, such as oppositional defiance disorder, conduct disorder, and academic and social difficulties. Adolescent girls with ADHD may be at higher risk for eating disorders than boys, although this difference tends to decrease by young adulthood.

SO, WHAT IS ADHD?

Ok, so we've debunked the myths associated with ADHD and established what it's not; let's look more closely at what it is. ADHD stands for Attention Deficit Hyperactivity Disorder, a neurodevelopmental disorder that typically begins in childhood and can continue into adulthood. While most cases are diagnosed in children under 12, someone can be diagnosed later in childhood or even as an adult if it was not recognized earlier.

ADHD symptoms are typically observed early in life and may become more apparent during significant changes, such as the start of formal schooling. It is characterized by inattention, hyperactivity, and impulsivity symptoms, which can transform a person's daily life, including social interactions, academic performance, and job productivity. Although symptoms of ADHD tend to improve with age, many individuals diagnosed with the condition during childhood may continue to experience difficulties as adults. People with ADHD are also at risk of experiencing other issues, such as sleep disorders and anxiety.

CAUSES OF ADHD

ADHD is a complex disorder whose exact causes are not yet fully understood, but it is believed to result from genetic and environmental factors. Let's zoom in on these risk factors.

Genetics

ADHD is believed to have a strong genetic component, with inherited genes from parents being a significant factor in its development. But the exact way in which ADHD is inherited is likely to be complex and is not believed to be linked to a single genetic mutation or defect. Research has shown that individuals with a family history of ADHD are more likely to develop the condition. This risk is higher among parents and siblings of individuals with ADHD.

Brain function and structure

Differences in the brains of people with ADHD have been identified by research, although the exact significance of these differences remains unclear. Brain scans have revealed that certain regions of the brain may be smaller in people with ADHD while other regions may be larger. Other studies have suggested that individuals with ADHD may have an imbalance in the neurotransmitters in the brain or that these chemicals may not function properly. We will discuss this in more detail subsequently.

Groups at risk

People who are most at risk of developing ADHD include:

- Individuals who were born prematurely (before the 37th week of pregnancy) or with low birth weight
- Maternal substance use during pregnancy (smoking, alcohol, or drug abuse) has been suggested as a potential risk factor for ADHD
- Those with epilepsy
- Individuals who have experienced brain damage either in the womb or after a severe head injury later in life are believed to be at higher risk of developing ADHD

It's worth noting that ADHD can affect individuals of any intellectual ability, but it appears to be more prevalent among those with learning difficulties.

THE NEUROSCIENCE OF THE ADHD BRAIN

Individuals with ADHD have been found to have lower levels of the neurotransmitter norepinephrine, which is closely associated with dopamine and stems from it. Dopamine helps regulate the brain's pleasure and reward center. Low levels of norepinephrine can lead to ADHD, which is why it can be used as a medication for this condition.

Four functional regions of the brain have impaired activity in individuals with ADHD, which are (Silver, 2023):

- The Frontal Cortex - controls high-level functions such as attention, executive function, and organization
- The Limbic System - located deeper in the brain, regulates emotions and attention
- The Basal Ganglia - when deficient, can cause inter-brain communication and information to "short-circuit," resulting in inattention or impulsivity
- The Reticular Activating System - is the major relay system among the many pathways that enter and leave the brain. A deficiency here can cause inattention, impulsivity, or hyperactivity

THE ADHD BRAIN VS. A NEUROTYPICAL BRAIN

Key differences in the brain of people with ADHD and those without relate to brain structure, function, and development. Individuals with ADHD may exhibit slower or distinct activity levels in certain brain areas compared to a neurotypical brain.

Brain structure

I briefly alluded to this earlier, and now I will expand on this more. Children with ADHD tend to have smaller brains than children who don't have ADHD, but this isn't an indication of intelligence. Volume differences exist in the amygdala and hippocampus, associated with motivation, memory, and emotion regulation. In children with ADHD, their brain matures slower. The frontal lobe's cognitive, attentional, and planning control regions show significant delays. On the other hand, the motor cortex developed faster than usual, which may account for symptoms such as restlessness and fidgeting.

The frontal lobe is responsible for cognitive functions such as attention, impulse control, and social behavior. People with ADHD may experience slower maturation in certain areas of this lobe, leading to dysfunction in cognitive skills. The premotor and prefrontal cortex, which are parts of the frontal lobe, engage in motor activity and attentional capacity. Individuals with ADHD may exhibit reduced activity in these brain regions.

Brain function

The subtle abnormalities in the brain structure and function of a person with ADHD can be seen through an X-ray or MRI. People with ADHD may not have enough computational capacity to handle the cognitive demands of a task. A link has been found by researchers between heightened functional connectivity in specific brain regions and clinical symptoms such as hyperactivity and restlessness. This suggests that inefficiencies in the processing of brain networks could be a potential explanation for some symptoms associated with ADHD. The condition can affect executive functioning skills related to:

- Attention
- Focus
- Concentration
- Memory
- Impulsivity
- Hyperactivity
- Organization
- Social skills
- Decision-making
- Planning
- motivation
- task-switching
- learning from past mistakes

Brain development

Individuals with ADHD may experience delays in the development of their brain networks, which could result in less efficient communication of specific messages, behaviors, or information. These brain networks may exhibit differences in functionality concerning focus, movement, and reward.

SYMPTOMS, DIAGNOSIS, AND TREATMENT

Symptoms in adults and children may differ. Symptoms can present in three ways:

1. Combined Presentation - If an individual displays sufficient symptoms of both inattention and hyperactivity-impulsivity criteria for the past six months.
2. Predominantly Inattentive Presentation - Symptoms of inattention, but not hyperactivity-impulsivity, were present for the past six months.
3. Predominantly Hyperactive-Impulsive Presentation -If enough symptoms of hyperactivity-impulsivity, but not inattention, were present for the past six months.

Symptoms in children

The symptoms of ADHD can be divided into two categories of behavioral issues - inattentiveness and hyperactivity/impulsiveness. In children and teenagers, the primary indications of inattentiveness include:

- Having a brief attention span and being easily sidetracked
- Displaying negligence, such as in schoolwork
- Appearing forgetful or misplacing things
- Being incapable of committing to tedious or time-consuming tasks
- Struggling to follow or execute instructions
- Continuously changing between activities or tasks
- Finding it challenging to organize tasks

Indicators of hyperactivity in children and teenagers include:

- Difficulty remaining seated, particularly in peaceful or tranquil environments
- Constant fidgeting or restlessness
- Difficulty focusing on tasks
- Excessive physical activity
- Excessive talking
- Inability to wait for their turn
- Acting without forethought
- Interrupting conversations
- Limited or no awareness of danger

Symptoms in adults

In adults, ADHD symptoms have been linked to the following:

- Inattentiveness and a lack of attention to detail
- A tendency to start new tasks without finishing old ones
- Poor organizational skills
- Difficulty focusing or prioritizing tasks
- Frequent misplacing or losing of items
- Forgetfulness
- Restlessness and feeling on edge
- Difficulty controlling impulses to speak out of turn or stay quiet
- Interrupting others while speaking and blurting out responses
- Mood swings, irritability, and a short temper
- Difficulty managing stress
- Extreme impatience
- Engaging in risky activities with little concern for personal safety or the safety of others, such as reckless driving

Related conditions in adults with ADHD

Similar to children and teenagers with ADHD, adults with ADHD may experience several related issues or conditions. Depression is a prevalent condition that often accompanies

ADHD in adults. Adults with ADHD may also have personality disorders, such as bipolar disorder, which cause significant differences in thinking, perception, emotion, or interpersonal relationships. Bipolar disorder involves mood swings from one extreme to another, and obsessive-compulsive disorder (OCD), which causes obsessive thoughts and compulsive behavior, are other conditions that adults with ADHD may experience. And the behavioral difficulties associated with ADHD can lead to social interaction and relationship challenges.

Diagnosis

To diagnose ADHD, healthcare providers must adhere to the American Psychiatric Association's Diagnostic and Statistical Manual, Fifth Edition (DSM-5) guidelines. By using this diagnostic criterion, individuals with ADHD can receive the proper diagnosis and treatment they require. According to the DSM-5, for children up to the age of 16, the diagnostic criterion for inattention requires six or more symptoms, while adolescents aged 17 and above and adults need to have five or more symptoms. These symptoms must have been present for at least six months and are considered inappropriate for the individual's developmental level. These are the same symptoms discussed earlier - inattentiveness and hyperactivity and their associated indicators. Additionally, the following criteria must be satisfied:

1. The presence of multiple inattentive or hyperactive-impulsive symptoms before the age of 12 years.
2. The occurrence of these symptoms in at least two settings, such as home, school, or work, and with friends or relatives.
3. The evidence shows that these symptoms interfere with or diminish the quality of social, academic, or occupational functioning.
4. The symptoms cannot be better explained by another mental disorder, such as a mood disorder, anxiety disorder, dissociative disorder, or personality disorder. Furthermore, the symptoms cannot be solely attributed to the presence of schizophrenia or another psychotic disorder.

Diagnosis in adults

For individuals aged 17 and above, the diagnostic criteria for ADHD require only five symptoms instead of six, as is necessary for younger children. Symptoms of ADHD may manifest differently in older individuals. For instance, hyperactivity in adults may present as excessive restlessness or causing fatigue in others due to their constant activity.

Treatment

Although there is no cure for ADHD, there are effective strategies for managing symptoms. Appropriate educational support, parental guidance, and medication, if necessary, for children can be helpful.

1. Medication

For adults with ADHD, medication is commonly the initial treatment option, but psychological therapies such as cognitive-behavioral therapy (CBT) can also be used. It's important to note the following:

- Medication for adult ADHD is more of a tool than a cure. ADHD medication is more effective when combined with other treatments that address emotional and behavioral issues.
- Everyone's response to ADHD medication is different. Some people may experience a drastic improvement, while others may really find that much relief. Finding the appropriate medication and dosage takes time since people have varying responses.
- ADHD medication should be monitored. Close monitoring of side effects and regular assessments of your well-being by you and your doctor are necessary to make necessary adjustments to the dosage. Without careful monitoring, ADHD medication becomes less effective and riskier.
- If you're on ADHD medication, it doesn't mean you'll always be on it. In case of unsatisfactory results, you may opt to discontinue ADHD medication safely. Yet inform your doctor of your decision and collaborate with them to gradually reduce your medication intake.

- Treatment is not always medication. Any action you take towards managing your symptoms is treatment, such as cognitive behavioral therapy.

2. Regular exercise

Engaging in physical activity helps to dissipate surplus energy that may cause impulsiveness. Moreover, it promptly increases the brain's dopamine, norepinephrine, and serotonin levels, which are all crucial in influencing focus and attention.

3. Importance of sleep

Enhancing your sleep quality can have a significant impact. Establishing a consistent sleep routine is crucial because inadequate sleep quality exacerbates ADHD symptoms. For better sleep, have a set sleep time and stick to it; keep your room dark and devoid of light, even the one from your devices; avoid taking caffeine later in the day; have a quiet time before going to bed; and talk to your doctor if your medication is keeping you up.

4. Eating right

Most nutritional challenges faced by adults with ADHD stem from impulsive behaviors and inadequate planning. To address this, it's important to cultivate mindfulness around your dietary habits. This means creating a meal plan, purchasing wholesome ingredients, scheduling regular mealtimes, and preparing food ahead of time to avoid becoming ravenously hungry. Keeping nutritious and convenient snacks readily available can prevent indulging in unhealthy vending machine snacks or fast-food meals. Schedule meals and snacks no more than 3 hours apart; cut back on sugar and caffeine; avoid junk food; and include sufficient omega-3 fatty acids, zinc, magnesium, iron, protein, and carbohydrates in your diet.

5. Therapy

Professionals trained in ADHD can provide valuable assistance in acquiring new coping mechanisms to manage symptoms and overcome problematic habits. They offer various therapies tailored to your specific needs, including stress and anger management, impulse control, time and money management, and organizational skills enhancement.

IT'S DIFFERENT FOR WOMEN

There's evidence to suggest that ADHD is more influential on women than it is on their male counterparts. The lived experience of women with ADHD suggests that the symptoms are different in women.

How symptoms differ in young women with ADHD

Despite having fewer DSM-5 symptoms, women with ADHD face similar levels of impairment as males with ADHD but are less likely to receive a diagnosis. ADHD is often diagnosed three times more in boys than girls. This means that girls can carry symptoms that can impact their lives without even knowing what it is.

Coping mechanisms

Research indicates that women with ADHD exhibit unique characteristics such as low self-esteem, challenges forming peer relationships, co-existing anxiety, and depression. Females with ADHD mask their feeling of underachievement and performance issues through coping strategies; they internalize their symptoms, experiencing anxiety, depression, and difficulties in emotional regulation.

Hormonal influence

During the development and onset of puberty in young girls, hormones play a crucial role in the symptoms associated with ADHD. The monthly fluctuations in estrogen and progesterone levels can affect the severity and manifestation of ADHD symptoms. ADHD symptoms tend to worsen with premenstrual symptoms due to the drop in hormone levels during the monthly cycle. These symptoms can be dismissed as 'that time of the month,' This can also be mislabeled at menopause when lower estrogen levels cause sleep, memory, and concentration impairment.

Sex norms and gender stereotypes

Gender norms and stereotypes can impact how women with ADHD perceive their symptoms and how others categorize their coping mechanisms. For example, inattentiveness could be labeled as talkative in the classroom. As women grow older, they often feel pressured to fit into societal expectations of being neat, organized, and well-behaved. These standards can feel unattainable, leaving women feeling inadequate and constantly struggling to keep up. This can lead to stress and unpredictability as women try to manage their impulses while feeling like they don't measure up. Unlike men with ADHD, women often feel compelled to hide their symptoms and develop coping mechanisms to mask their struggles. This can create a constant sense of tension and feelings of inadequacy, which can be difficult to articulate or understand without a proper diagnosis.

The diagnostic gap for women with ADHD

A complex issue among children with ADHD is that boys are more prone than girls to co-occurring disorders that lead to being identified as requiring assistance. It is frequent to observe learning disabilities and behavioral disorders such as oppositional defiant disorder, which typically demand significant resources and attention.

ADHD diagnosis in women typically occurs during their thirties, with many identifying their own symptoms after observing them in their children. Ongoing research on gender differences in ADHD presentation has prompted efforts to improve screening methods and standards, reducing the number of undiagnosed young girls in schools.

Despite these efforts, many women worldwide remain undiagnosed, lacking an understanding of the root causes of their difficulties. Proper diagnostic procedures and treatment plans are crucial for these women to achieve the quality of life they deserve.

WHAT ADHD LOOKS LIKE IN WOMEN

We've established that ADHD is more likely to go undiagnosed in women, who are also more prone to the inattentive type of the disorder. Women may develop coping mechanisms, including internalization, because of certain gender norms. But the question remains; how does ADHD affect the day-to-day life of an adult woman? Let's look at some of these unique struggles.

Relationships

Symptoms of ADHD can have subtle or obvious effects on relationships. Adult women with ADHD may feel inadequate in relationships that don't align with traditional female stereotypes. Relationships may suffer due to chronic disorganization and forgetfulness. Undiagnosed adult ADHD can bring feelings of inadequacy and comparison against standards that don't highlight individual strengths. To improve relationships with yourself and others, learning self-compassion and navigating your strengths and weaknesses is essential.

Work or school life

Women with ADHD often experience hyperfocus on topics of interest while finding uninteresting or tedious tasks challenging and uncomfortable to engage with. This can make shifting attention between different projects difficult, leading to negative labels such as "lazy" or "careless" when tasks are incomplete. It is not uncommon to have an untidy workspace, incomplete projects, or missed deadlines in daily life. Undiagnosed ADHD can also lead to missing out on well-deserved promotions or recognition. Individuals with ADHD can also experience perfectionism in work or school, which can cause them to overcompensate for their challenges by overachieving, which can be mentally and physically draining.

Daily tasks

Daily tasks can feel overwhelming and daunting when living with ADHD, leading to feelings of being stuck or overwhelmed by everyday life. Seeing others easily complete these tasks while you struggle can be frustrating. Additionally, women with ADHD may find it challenging to relax and often take on multiple projects without seeing them through to completion, leaving them feeling like they are not making progress in life.

Many women with ADHD spend much time cleaning up messes and feel they are not reaching their goals. They sometimes feel their untidy environment is a reflection of who they are. Even simple chores can turn into lengthy distractions, resulting in a feeling of moving in circles and not achieving one's potential. It can be difficult to redirect focus from engaging activities or topics back to mundane tasks in daily life.

MENTAL HEALTH CONDITIONS THAT COMMONLY OCCUR WITH ADHD IN ADULT WOMEN

Co-morbid conditions can occur alongside ADHD. The presence of these conditions can sometimes obscure or worsen symptoms of ADHD, which can make obtaining an accurate diagnosis tougher. Some of these conditions include:

Substance abuse disorder

Women with ADHD may experience an increased likelihood of developing substance use disorders due to factors such as chronic stress, feelings of being misunderstood, under-stimulation, and impulsivity. Substance abuse or addiction, including drugs or alcohol, is often used to cope with low self-esteem and feelings of inadequacy commonly associated with ADHD in women.

Anxiety disorder

Women with ADHD often experience comorbidities such as Social Anxiety, Obsessive-Compulsive Disorder, Separation Anxiety Disorder, and Generalized Anxiety Disorder. It is estimated that approximately 50% of adults with ADHD also have an accompanying anxiety disorder.

Mood disorders

ADHD is often comorbid with depressive disorders like Major Depressive Disorder, Seasonal Affective Disorder, and Bipolar Disorder. The symptoms of mood disorders, such as irritability, may overlap with ADHD, showing how important it is to obtain a diagnosis from a professional trained in identifying both conditions.

Eating disorders

The incidence of eating disorders, particularly Bulimia Nervosa, is higher in women with ADHD. The severity of certain ADHD symptoms, such as impulsivity, appears to have an adverse impact on the manifestation of eating disorders. Women with ADHD are also more prone to engage in disordered eating behaviors like binging and extreme dieting, with or without developing a full-blown eating disorder.

Other disorders in adult ADHD in women

Along with the comorbidities mentioned above, other challenges like sleep disorders (like insomnia and narcolepsy) and personality disorders can also accompany ADHD. The good news is that many effective treatment options are available to minimize symptoms and enhance the quality of life. But a crucial first step is seeking a diagnosis and collaborating with a healthcare professional on a treatment plan.

SUMMARY

In this chapter, we have explored understanding:

- What ADHD is
- The causes of ADHD are unclear, but it is believed to result from a combination of genetic and environmental factors
- How ADHD can be misdiagnosed in women due to masking
- The size, function, and development of an ADHD brain are different from a neurotypical brain
- Medication is just a tool and a cure for ADHD
- ADHD can be managed with diet, exercise, sleep, medication, and therapy
- ADHD affects women differently than it does men
- Some co-occurring mental health conditions can happen alongside ADHD, such as mood disorder, anxiety disorder, and an eating disorder

Now that we've debunked some myths and fully understood what ADHD is, I'm sure you can agree with me that ADHD is not that bad. It is a condition that can be managed if correctly diagnosed. Let's take a deeper dive into why ADHD isn't that bad.

2

ADHD IS NOT SO BAD

IT'S NOT SO BAD AFTERALL - INSIDE AVA'S HEAD

I've been feeling pretty down lately. I was diagnosed with ADHD, which blew my mind because I'm a woman in my 30s, and I had no idea I had ADHD all my life. It was not until yesterday that I got my pick-me-up. I read the most inspirational story and feel like a new person today! I feel like, finally! Someone understands. The story is about a woman who struggled with ADHD, motor tics, and bullying from a young age. She constantly felt trapped in an invisible bubble, and doctors dismissed her condition as anxiety. She tried to fit in as a child and copied her friends to blend in. She became interested in psychology to figure out what was wrong with her and tried hard to control her emotions and avoid social conflict.

In university, she faced new challenges, such as a lack of focus, a lack of organization, and the inability to follow her classes. She was met with judgment and criticism from her peers and professors, which took a toll on her self-esteem. Despite her hard work and effort, she struggled with the basics due to a neurological condition called aphantasia. She could not create a mental image, and she didn't have a visual memory. She tried to adapt by creating a new process and a list of steps to recreate drawings.

After getting her degree, the woman was constantly exhausted, overwhelmed, and unmotivated. Eventually, she met another neurodivergent who instantly recognized her condition, and they both found solace in each other's company. They both faced oppression from most neurotypical people who judged their characters based on their inability to perform simple tasks or conform to the neurotypical way of seeing the world.

This incredible woman eventually became a doctor, despite her struggles with ADHD. She was too focused on her diagnosis and the internalized ableism from society's judgment. But meeting another neurodivergent person helped dispel this ableism, and she learned to accept herself for who she was. She now advocates for neurodiversity and strives to help others with similar conditions.

Mind blown! This story spoke to me in chapters and volumes. It's like I recognize myself in her. Most of her struggles are nothing new to me; I'm in the choir! What excited me most was how she managed to do something she loved despite the challenges and obstacles. It just helped me see that ADHD is not so bad after all. It's all the trappings of an ableist society!

THINGS TO LOVE ABOUT YOUR ADHD

Make no mistake; your ADHD is no burden. It makes you the unique individual you are, and you're worth celebrating. Recognize that your ADHD represents distinctive qualities and skills that set you apart, making you more innovative, spontaneous, compassionate, and enthusiastic than most people. I will share with you some of the top reasons you should unwaveringly, all-in love your ADHD.

The drive of ADHD hyperfocus

The trademark hyperfocus that comes with ADHD is a huge plus when you channel all your attention and energy into meaningful work. Many scientists, writers, and artists with ADHD have achieved remarkable success in their careers, largely owing to their capacity to concentrate on their work for extended periods.

Real ADHD resilience

Granted, ADHD can be challenging and is not always easy to manage. You've likely experienced your fair share of setbacks and awkward moments throughout your life (or at least you might know someone who has). However, you have the innate ability to persevere through difficulties, adjust your approaches when needed, and problem-solve even the most intricate issues. You can find hope in difficult situations and are able to recover after falling down, maintaining a positive outlook even when faced with challenges.

A people person

People with ADHD often exhibit qualities such as brightness, creativity, and a sense of humor. But you already know this; you're all these awesome things. Despite facing difficulties, you've discovered innovative strategies to cope with your symptoms and have cultivated humility and self-esteem. Taken together, these traits make you a delight to interact with!

Generosity and empathy

People with ADHD exhibit empathy towards others and tend to be kind and generous in their actions. I'm pretty sure you've heard these great things about yourself from friends or family. Whether it's by offering a listening ear to a friend in need, helping others without being asked, or sharing your last cookie with a stranger, you often go out of your way to show kindness to those around you, going above and beyond to make them feel loved and supported.

Your empathetic nature stems from your heightened sensitivity to the emotions of others, which enables you to understand and relate to the feelings of those around you. Most individuals with ADHD tend to have an intense desire for social connections and may go to great lengths to form and maintain meaningful relationships with others. Whether through small acts of kindness or larger gestures, you have the unique ability to touch the lives of those around you and positively impact the world.

Ingenious thinking

As we've already established, ADHD comes with its unique brand of creativity that allows those who have it to approach tasks and solve problems in ingenious and innovative ways. You may approach problems from a different angle than others, but this often results in highly effective and unexpected solutions. You often find a system that works for you as an individual, whether it's a traditional method or a personalized one.

A strong sense of fairness

Whether through personal experience of living with accommodations or struggling without them, individuals with ADHD recognize that fairness and equality are not always the same thing. They understand that neurodivergent individuals have unique needs to thrive and are dedicated to supporting anyone who may benefit from their assistance. Their commitment to helping others is driven by their own experiences and the empathy that they have developed through navigating their own challenges. They are often advocates for neurodiversity and work to educate others about the different ways in which individuals with ADHD and other neurodivergent conditions may need support. Individuals with ADHD are dedicated to creating a more inclusive and supportive world, one that recognizes and celebrates the diversity of all individuals, including those with unique ways of thinking and processing information.

They understand that success is not a one-size-fits-all approach.

Willingness to take a risk

It is believed that Thomas Edison, a renowned inventor, may have had ADHD. Despite facing seemingly insurmountable obstacles, he dedicated all his efforts towards inventing the light bulb. His perseverance paid off, and his triumph was incredibly sweet because he had to take risks and face countless failures to achieve it. Edison's story is a reminder that you can do whatever you put your mind to.

Spontaneity

Sometimes, impulsive actions can lead to marvelous outcomes. We all enjoy the unplanned moments and adventures that keep life interesting and individuals with ADHD excel in this area. That's one of the things I absolutely love about ADHD. There's no overthinking; you just do it. Individuals with ADHD can channel their impulsiveness into spontaneity, which may make them the center of attention in social gatherings or more adventurous and willing to step out of their comfort zones and challenge the norm.

A great sense of humor

Individuals with ADHD who have adapted well have developed the ability to use humor as a coping mechanism in challenging situations, alleviating stress, enhancing relationships, influencing perspectives, and accomplishing various other goals.

Constant surprises

Stumbling upon forgotten items such as money or a tasty treat can transform life into a series of delightful surprises, leaving you wondering what other treasures may be waiting to be uncovered. For a person with ADHD, it's surprises galore!

Last of the romantics

Individuals with ADHD bring increased vigor to their romantic encounters. They often exhibit exuberant displays of affection towards their partners and maintain a steadfast belief in the power of love, even during periods of difficulty in their relationships. I love that.

Engaging conversational skills

There's no doubt about it; having ADHD means you'll never experience a dull moment! Your mind is constantly buzzing, prompting you to explore new ideas and ask thought-provoking questions. Awkward silences in conversation are practically unheard of!

Compassion

Individuals with ADHD are often super kind-hearted and always ready to help a friend in need. They have a special knack for showing empathy and understanding towards others, which makes them great listeners and fantastic companions. You can count on them to be there for you, no matter what, and they'll always lend a hand when you need it most. So, if you have a buddy with ADHD, hold onto them tight because they're sure to be one of the most caring and compassionate people in your life!

Persistence

The ability to persist through difficulties is a superpower in itself, hands down. This is something you can expect to find in people with ADHD. They set their sights on something and get it done. It's remarkable because despite the difficulties faced, they still have the tenacity to persist and come out on the other side.

Superstar creativity

Superstar, check; creativity, check. People diagnosed with ADHD often possess exceptional intelligence and creativity. Case in point, Justin Timberlake, Adam Levine, Simone Biles, and Alexis Hernandez. Their superstar creativity has taken them to the world stage.

Advocacy

So often, when ADHD is misunderstood, people with the condition can help clarify it because they have lived it. Personally, I would much rather hear it from someone who has firsthand experience than someone who only has theories.

Contagious motivation

Let's be honest, high energy is contagious. People with ADHD inspire others with their passion, drive, and out-of-the-box thinking. They are like beacons of light that draw people into pursuing their own goals.

WOMEN WITH ADHD WHO ROCK

Women with ADHD are straight-up warriors. They fight tooth and nail just to get their symptoms checked out, diagnosed, and treated. On top of that, they're dealing with a world that's pretty much all about guys. Let's look at some truly amazing women who show you, you can come out on top and crush it!

Roxy Olin

Roxy Olin, who appears in reality TV shows like The City and The Hills, has struggled with ADHD since childhood. She was prescribed Ritalin, but it didn't work for her. As a teenager, she was formally diagnosed with ADHD and started taking Adderall. When she entered a rehab program that didn't allow her to take the medication, she struggled and got into multiple car accidents. Her therapist advocated for her and helped her learn time-management tricks to succeed in her career. Olin uses strategies to stay organized, and she discusses her ADHD openly in relationships, knowing it's a part of who she is.

Robin Stephens

Robin Stephens, a professional organizer with Your Life in Order, has been diagnosed with ADHD and bipolar disorder. She was drawn to the job because she couldn't function or concentrate in a cluttered environment. She struggled to sit still in class as a child and was a perfectionist. After being diagnosed with bipolar disorder, she learned about the link between it and ADHD. Now, she uses strategies like to-do lists and breaking down tasks into manageable chunks to manage her symptoms. Robin talks quickly and has boundless energy, which can affect her dating life, but she has learned to accept herself just as she is.

Evelyn Polk-Green

Evelyn Polk-Green, a former president of ADDA and a project director at Illinois STAR Net, has ADHD and sees it as an advantage. She was successful at work, managing several projects at the same time, but couldn't keep her house in order. After reading about ADHD, she finally understood that she was also coping with the disorder. She now takes medication to be productive and advises other women with ADHD to figure out how the disorder affects them and use their strengths to overcome their weaknesses.

Katherine Ellison

Pulitzer Prize-winning journalist Katherine Ellison always knew she wanted to be a writer. After struggling with inconsistency in her work and seeking therapy, she was diagnosed with ADHD at age 49, following her oldest son's diagnosis. She has since tried various treatments, including metacognition, neurofeedback, meditation, exercise, and medication. Katherine believes that accepting her condition and finding her passion are keys to managing her ADHD. Her book 'Buzz: A Year of Paying Attention' chronicles her experiences of connecting with her son, who also has ADHD.

Cynthia Gerdes

Cynthia Gerdes, the owner of an award-winning restaurant in Minneapolis, credits her ADHD for her entrepreneurial success, saying that it's easy to do a million things at once. Despite the long hours her jobs demanded, she found herself lost in smaller tasks like grocery shopping. When she found out she had ADHD, she finally understood why she had more energy than everyone else. Gerdes has found that adjusting her schedule is enough to keep her ADHD in check, such as taking breaks during meetings. However, she still struggles with grocery shopping and relies on her chef husband for support.

Patricia Quinn

Dr. Patricia Quinn, a medical practitioner based in Washington, D.C., believes it is possible to use ADHD to become successful. Quinn was diagnosed with ADHD in 1972 while researching the condition, which often goes undiagnosed in girls and women. She believes that her hyperfocus and impulsivity, which were initially seen as challenges, are qualities that have helped her become successful in her medical career. Quinn's mission is to highlight the issues facing women and girls with ADHD and has co-founded 'The National Center for Girls and Women with ADHD.'

Sari Solden

Sari Solden is an expert on ADHD's effect on women and has struggled with ADHD herself. She understands the shame and stigma women with ADHD experience when they struggle to stay organized, maintain friendships, and keep a tidy home. After recognizing her symptoms as an attention deficit and receiving a diagnosis from a doctor, Solden felt liberated. She now works in private practice. Finding and working with other women with ADHD has helped Solden and inspired her to continue her work.

YOU ARE NOT THE SUM OF IT ALL

Many people assume ADHD is a personal flaw rather than a neurological disorder. If you have ADHD, you've likely experienced this first-hand. People may blame you for your symptoms, suggest that you simply need to try harder, or believe that you can overcome your challenges through sheer willpower alone. But these beliefs are uninformed. Your symptoms are not your fault, and just as you didn't choose to have ADHD, you cannot will those symptoms away. It's important to note that constant criticism, blame, and shame will not alleviate ADHD symptoms but may contribute to a drop in self-esteem.

How ADHD can affect self-esteem and how to cultivate self-worth

ADHD can significantly impact an individual's self-esteem. Your challenges when you have ADHD make it difficult to meet your own expectations and those of others. This can lead to feelings of inadequacy, shame, and low self-worth.

Self-esteem vs. self-worth

You've probably used these two terms interchangeably because they do sound like one and the same, right? While closely connected, these two don't carry identical meanings. Self-esteem is often inclusive of your talents, capabilities, personality traits, and achievements. This perception of yourself may vary based on the events occurring in your life and the feedback received from others. In contrast, self-worth is a gauge of self-value as an individual, encompassing feelings of self-assuredness, desirability, and worthiness of admiration and esteem from others.

The connection between ADHD and self-esteem

Consistently, it has been found that people with ADHD have lower self-esteem than their neurotypical counterparts. There are a few reasons for this:

- **Stigma** - ADHD can carry a social stigma as it's not always recognized as a severe condition like other mental health issues and chronic illnesses. Individuals with ADHD may face discrimination from those around them, potentially leading to a decreased sense of self-esteem from recurring rejection.
- **Lack of accommodation** - People with ADHD often struggle to get the necessary accommodations to succeed in school and work. Difficulties with organization and time management can lead to low grades and poor reviews, which can mask their innate talents. Lower grades in school can limit choices of college or employment, leading to a lack of opportunities to find an environment that suits their thinking style. This can lead to a skewed perception of their abilities and an underestimation of their full potential.
- **Criticism** - A survey found that people with ADHD were most often criticized for behaviors related to focus, forgetfulness, organization, and time management, which are all largely outside their control. ADHD affects how the brain processes time, making it difficult to stick to a schedule or plan things in sequence. Criticism of ADHD symptoms can feel like a personal attack and can damage self-esteem.

- **Rejection sensitivity** - People with ADHD may be especially sensitive to rejection, which can make them perceive neutral comments as criticism and react strongly to them. Some individuals with ADHD also experience rejection-sensitive dysphoria (RSD), which can lead to panic, rage, or guilt in response to even mildly negative comments. RSD can also cause individuals to berate themselves or feel self-loathing at the thought of disappointing others.

How to boost self-esteem

Given all these potential challenges, you might wonder how to push back against feelings of insecurity and self-doubt. Here's a good place to start:

- People with ADHD often struggle to complete tasks, which can lead to a sense of failure and low self-esteem. To increase self-esteem, break tasks into smaller, manageable steps and celebrate progress along the way.
- ADHD can also affect social skills, leading to difficulties in forming and maintaining relationships. To build self-esteem, focus on your strengths, and seek out social situations that play to your strengths.
- People with ADHD may doubt their abilities and feel like they don't measure up to their peers. To boost self-esteem, focus on your strengths and accomplishments, and practice self-compassion.

- People with ADHD may engage in negative self-talk, criticizing themselves for their shortcomings. To increase self-esteem, practice positive self-talk and challenge negative beliefs about yourself.
- People with ADHD may feel overwhelmed by daily tasks, leading to feelings of stress and anxiety. To build self-esteem, practice stress-management techniques, such as mindfulness, exercise, and deep breathing.

If you are a parent of a child with ADHD, your behavior can greatly impact their self-esteem by

- Acknowledging their strengths
- Setting them up to succeed by giving them the tools to do it well
- Avoid comparing your child to neurotypical kids
- Saving discipline for the things your kid does on purpose, not the ones they can't help
- Show them plenty of affection

It's important to remember that ADHD does not define who you are as a person. By focusing on your strengths, cultivating self-compassion, and practicing self-care, you can build your self-esteem and overcome the challenges of ADHD. Seeking a therapist or counselor's help who specializes in ADHD can also be a helpful resource.

Undiagnosed ADHD can affect self-esteem, too

Undiagnosed ADHD can make individuals even more vulnerable. A study showed that adults with undiagnosed ADHD symptoms scored an average of 3 points lower on the Rosenberg Self-Esteem Scale than those with a diagnosis. Without an explanation for their struggles, individuals may assume they are naturally messy or lazy. However, a diagnosis can help avoid self-blame and criticism and find the right support.

When to get professional support

Although there is no pill that can instantly improve self-esteem, therapy is a helpful tool for not only managing ADHD symptoms but also cultivating a healthier relationship with yourself. The combination of ADHD and low self-esteem can lead to distinct challenges in daily life. Seeking therapy may be beneficial for the following reasons:

- Find yourself censoring your conversations due to fear of annoying others
- Put yourself down when feeling frustrated or guilty
- Worry about being disliked when someone doesn't respond to your texts or match your enthusiasm
- Have a history of bullying or abuse
- Lose motivation to engage in basic self-care activities like bathing and eating

If your child has ADHD and often puts themselves down to garner laughter from others, reacts to compliments with suspicion or irritation, avoids trying new things out of fear of failure and embarrassment, becomes upset or angry when asked to perform seemingly easy tasks like cleaning their room, or expresses confusion or frustration about being excluded from friend groups, it may be beneficial to connect them with a therapist.

HOW TO REGAIN YOUR CONFIDENCE

Research shows that a person's self-esteem rises over time and peaks by the time you're 60 years old, mainly due to professional success and financial security. But this might not be the case for adults with ADHD. As they enter middle age and approach retirement, self-confidence, and self-esteem decrease. As they age, people with ADHD tend to feel a sense of dissatisfaction and disappointment, viewing themselves as unsuccessful compared to their contemporaries. Despite years of attempting to change their behavior, they often experience a sense of hopelessness. Financial insecurity is also common due to inconsistent money management and a lack of long-term financial planning.

Manage ADHD symptoms

The foundation of a person's self-esteem lies in their core beliefs about themselves, which are influenced by how much they appreciate and like themselves. If a person struggles with ADHD and does not receive proper management, it can cause a constant state of frustration and self-criticism. The accumulation of negative experiences, such as real and perceived failures, self-blaming, guilt, and criticisms, can severely damage a person's self-esteem. Over time, a drop in self-esteem may lead to other serious problems like anxiety, substance abuse, mood disorders, and related mental health issues.

By effectively managing ADHD, you can prevent the erosion of self-esteem and reverse any emotional damage. Remembering that your past does not define you is essential, and that it is never too late to make positive changes. A robust treatment program, including medication, behavior therapy, ADHD coaching, and self-care practices such as exercise, healthy sleep, and good nutrition, can help in managing ADHD biology and behaviors reasonably well, breaking the cycle of frustration and feelings of failure.

Stop negative thinking

To break free from feeling stuck, people with ADHD must acknowledge, confront, and reject negative thoughts that are associated with and contribute to their low self-esteem. Although negative messages may feel like a natural part of life, you should not accept them as normal or healthy. Instead, view them as cognitive distortions that need to be addressed. Building stronger self-esteem is challenging, but it is a battle that you can win. Here are some techniques to help curb negative thinking and regain self-confidence:

- **Understand and accept your ADHD biology** and focus on adjusting your behavior. Reframe ADHD as a neutral characteristic and avoid attaching negative connotations to it. Labeling yourself or others with ADHD as broken can harm your self-esteem and sense of value. Start working to promote a more positive and accepting mindset.
- **ADHD is not a character defect** nor a disease to be cured. They're neurobiological symptoms that can be effectively managed with appropriate strategies and treatments.
- **It is never too late to learn to manage ADHD better.** Regardless of age, it is always possible to improve your ability to manage ADHD.
- **Identify and appreciate your accomplishments.** In case you find it challenging to accomplish this, consider seeking the honest feedback of two or three individuals who are familiar with you.
- **Assess your strengths and weaknesses.** If asking for feedback from those close to you is challenging, consider seeking input from external sources. Take time to acknowledge and value your strengths while setting practical and healthy goals for yourself. It's important to address areas of weakness. We all have them.
- **Identify, monitor, challenge, and dismiss your critical self-talk.** See it as a continuous struggle that must be fought until the end, no matter how long it

takes. With dedication and perseverance, it will gradually become less challenging. You can change negative self-talk by learning of this negative self-talk, challenging it, practicing positive self-talk, stepping outside of yourself, talking it out, shelving it, and focusing on the present.
- **Don't compare yourself to other people.** This isn't a great thing to do because it will get you to believe you're inferior, which is simply not true.
- **Focus on solutions, not problems**. When an issue comes up, ask yourself, "What actions can I take to address it?"
- **Get past the "could have done, should have done, would have done" scripts.** Don't dwell on the things you haven't accomplished. Instead, concentrate on the actions you can take each day going forward.

SUMMARY

In this chapter, we have learned:

- Above all, ADHD is not that bad at all
- See it as a superpower because of the unique characteristics it brings out in you, such as resilience, hyperfocus, and empathy
- There are great examples of amazing women who have ADHD and are excelling in their lives and careers

- ADHD is often misunderstood as a character flaw, which is not true
- You can share your experiences and help correct misinformation about ADHD
- ADHD can impact self-esteem and self-worth, especially when compared to neurotypical people
- You have every reason to feel confident and have bucketloads of self-esteem because you are unique and have a wonderful perspective on things
- If you are struggling with low self-esteem, see a therapist who can help you
- A really good way to manage ADHD symptoms is to stop negative thinking and self-talk and start having a more positive outlook

As we close off this chapter, I want to reiterate what an amazing, wonderfully made individual you are. Everything about you is great and your ADHD is not bad. You can do anything you set your mind to, and you can live a fulfilling and happy life, especially when you practice healthy living and self-care. Let us now turn our focus to health and self-care.

3

HEALTH & SELF-CARE

THE WEEK I'VE HAD!

I've had quite a week! I took on a few more clients, and now I feel like I'm drowning. The more stressed I get, the more I feel like eating. I'm such a terrible binge eater. This hasn't really done anything for me. Besides the guilt of taking in all that gunk, I just feel so unhappy and kinda depressed. I had a chat with my doctor, who explained how my eating and working habits were the culprits of my feeling the way I do. She told me to start eating healthier, cut out on unhealthy snacks, take up some exercise, and lessen my workload. I started a cycling class yesterday and cleared my snack cupboard. So far, so good. One foot in front of the other, right? I'm optimistic these changes will yield results.

YOUR LIFESTYLE WILL DETERMINE YOUR FUTURE

If you're an adult with ADHD or the spouse or parent of someone who does, you're likely familiar with the challenges that can come with this condition. It, therefore, goes without saying that looking out for yourself (or your significant other) is a top priority. I'm going to highlight some lifestyle changes and daily habits that will help you lead a healthy, functional, and more satisfying life with ADHD.

- Build an ADHD-friendly group that understands the challenges you face
- Build brain-healthy daily habits
- Get a good night's sleep
- Adopt brain-friendly nutrition
- Harness the power of exercise
- Practice stress management
- Create an ADHD-friendly environment

GET ENOUGH SLEEP

Approximately 25% to 50% of individuals with ADHD suffer from sleep difficulties, ranging from insomnia to secondary sleep conditions. Medical professionals increasingly acknowledge the significance of addressing sleep issues and the favorable effects that restful sleep can have on the quality of life of individuals with ADHD.

ADHD and sleep

People with ADHD are more prone to experiencing sleep problems beginning around puberty, including shorter sleep time, difficulty sleeping, and a higher risk of developing a sleep disorder. Individuals who exhibit mostly inattentive symptoms are more prone to having a later bedtime. On the other hand, individuals with predominantly hyperactive-impulsive symptoms are more likely to experience insomnia. Those with combined hyperactive-impulsive and inattentive ADHD tend to suffer from poor sleep quality and a delayed bedtime. The symptoms of ADHD often resemble those of sleep deprivation. These sleep problems can cause forgetfulness and difficulty concentrating during the day. In children, hyperactive and impulsive behaviors may be caused by fatigue, making it challenging to differentiate between whether these symptoms arise from ADHD or a lack of sleep. Consequently, this could lead to incorrect diagnoses or prevent the detection of sleep disorders.

The biology behind the ADHD-sleep connection

Some experts suggest that sleep problems associated with ADHD may stem from impaired arousal, alertness, and regulation circuits in the brain. Yet others propose that these sleep problems may be linked to a delayed circadian rhythm with a later onset of melatonin production. While some individuals may sleep easier with the calming effects of stimulant medications often prescribed for ADHD, these medications can harm many people. The presence of coexisting conditions, such as anxiety and depression, as well as inadequate sleep hygiene, are also likely to contribute to sleep problems.

How ADHD-related sleep problems affect daily life

People with both ADHD and sleep problems tend to experience a lower quality of life and report more severe ADHD symptoms. Chronic sleep deprivation can increase the likelihood of individuals experiencing depression, anxiety, hyperactivity, inattention, difficulty processing information, and a higher body mass index (BMI). Over time, prolonged sleep deprivation can make individuals more susceptible to developing physical health issues.

Experiencing daytime sleepiness can upend an individual's performance at school or work. For individuals with ADHD, being judged for sleeping at inappropriate times can be frustrating as it is a symptom of their condition and difficult to control. Furthermore, sudden bouts of sleepiness can be hazardous when operating machinery or performing activities that require alertness and concentration.

Poor sleep quality can cause daytime fatigue, resulting in individuals with ADHD feeling irritable, restless, grumpy, tired, and struggling to focus at school or work. These symptoms can be misinterpreted as a mood disorder. Children with ADHD with sleep problems may also be more prone to anxiety and behavioral difficulties. These sleep-related problems not only impact the individual with ADHD but also affect their families and caregivers. Research suggests that caregivers of children with ADHD and sleep problems are more likely to experience depression, anxiety, stress, and tardiness at their job.

Sleep disorders commonly found in people with ADHD

Individuals with ADHD are more prone to certain sleep disorders. Let's take a closer look.

Insomnia

Even individuals who are not typically hyperactive during the day may encounter racing thoughts and bursts of energy at night that impede their ability to fall asleep, resulting in insomnia. Nighttime can provide a perfect chance for some individuals to concentrate intensely on a task without disturbances. Even so, this makes it challenging to relax and settle down for the night, which can disrupt their sleep-wake cycle. As time passes, insomnia can exacerbate as people associate bedtime with stress.

Many individuals with ADHD suffer from daytime drowsiness and difficulty waking up due to poor sleep quality. Others may experience disturbed sleep with frequent awakenings, which do not refresh them.

Circadian rhythm sleep disorders

People with ADHD tend to be more alert during the evening, making it challenging to fulfill their work or school obligations. The presence of circadian rhythm sleep disorders in individuals with ADHD may be linked to a smaller pineal gland, disruptions in the internal body clock, and delayed melatonin release. Delayed sleep-wake phase disorder, also known as delayed sleep phase syndrome (DSPS), is a circadian rhythm sleep disorder often observed in individuals with ADHD. DSPS is characterized by a delay in the sleep-wake cycle of at least two hours, which can interfere with time-sensitive activities such as work or school. People with DSPS may find it difficult to fall asleep at night, leading to heightened exhaustion, disorientation, and reduced attentiveness the next day. To address DSPS, targeted melatonin supplements or bright light therapy can help regulate the sleep-wake cycle and alleviate its symptoms.

Sleep-disordered breathing

A third of individuals with ADHD experience sleep-disordered breathing (SDB), which entails snoring and sleep apnea. SDB can result in disrupted sleep and daytime sleepiness, often manifesting in symptoms resembling ADHD. Research suggests that in children, removing the tonsils may improve symptoms of ADHD and sleep apnea, while in adults, CPAP therapy is considered a more effective approach.

Restless legs syndrome

If you've got restless legs syndrome (RLS), you might feel tingling in your legs that can mess with your ability to doze off. Nearly 50% of people with ADHD also have RLS or other periodic limb movement disorders. If kids have both

ADHD and RLS, they may spend more time in light sleep stage 1, which isn't super restful. Experts think RLS might be linked to iron and dopamine deficiencies, often seen in people with ADHD.

Narcolepsy

People with narcolepsy tend to doze off during the day abruptly and may have trouble resting well at night. Interestingly, adults with narcolepsy are twice as likely to have shown signs of ADHD as kids. The connection between the two isn't exactly clear, but experts think that the sleepiness caused by narcolepsy could lead to ADHD symptoms. It's also possible that both conditions stem from the same source, like a gene or neurotransmitter issue. Narcolepsy is usually treated with medication.

Sleep Tips

Sleep interventions may help to improve sleep, ADHD symptoms, daily functioning, and behavior. To reinforce the connection between bed and sleep, children, adolescents, and adults with ADHD need to maintain a consistent bedtime routine and practice good sleep hygiene habits. Developing a personalized system that works for you may involve making gradual changes and tracking improvements over time. Some useful tips to consider include:

- Cut out sugar, caffeine, and alcohol intake a few hours before bedtime

- Avoid screen time an hour before bed
- Avoid stimulating activities and projects that require hyper-focusing in the evening
- Make the bed a stress-free zone
- Get enough exercise and sunlight during the day
- Develop a bedtime routine you enjoy, like reading, spending time with your pets, or taking a warm bath
- Keep the bedroom dark, cool, and quiet, and use a white noise machine if necessary
- Maintain a consistent sleep schedule - same bedtime and wake-up time daily
- Use a weighted blanket

HEALTHY EATING

Although there is no definitive scientific evidence that proves ADHD is caused by diet or nutritional problems, research suggests that some foods may affect symptom severity in a small subset of individuals. Consult your doctor before you make any changes to your diet, including eliminating certain foods or taking supplements. Although certain foods and supplements may alleviate symptoms of your condition, they may also interfere with your medication or its absorption.

What Is an ADHD diet?

Your diet and any dietary supplements you consume could impact the functionality of your brain and reduce symptoms like lack of concentration or restlessness. Ideally, your eating patterns should optimize brain function.

- **Overall nutrition.** Certain foods can either improve or worsen your symptoms. It is also possible that some foods you are not consuming could alleviate your symptoms.
- **Supplementation diets** entail adding vitamins, minerals, or other nutrients to your diet to compensate for any deficiencies that may result from inadequate intake through regular food consumption. Advocates of these diets suggest that if you are deficient in specific nutrients, it may exacerbate your symptoms.
- **Elimination diets** involve abstaining from certain foods or ingredients that you suspect may trigger certain behaviors or exacerbate your symptoms.

Eat nutritious food

According to experts, what's good for the brain is probably good for ADHD. This includes the following:

- **High-protein diet**. Some really good sources of protein include beans, cheese, eggs, meat, and nuts. Eat these foods in the morning and for after-school snacks. They may improve concentration and possibly extend the effects of ADHD medications.

- **More complex carbohydrates.** Eat vegetables and fruits, including oranges, tangerines, pears, grapefruit, apples, and kiwi. Eat these foods in the evening, and they may help improve sleep.
- **More omega-3 fatty acids.** Sources include tuna, salmon, and other cold-water white fish, walnuts, Brazil nuts, and olive and canola oils. Consider taking an omega-3 fatty acid supplement. The FDA approved an omega compound called Vayarin as part of an ADHD management strategy.

Foods to avoid

High-sugar foods and snacks

Studies suggest sugar may worsen ADHD symptoms. One study found that hyperactive children became more destructive and restless with higher sugar consumption. Another study showed that high-sugar diets increased inattention in some kids. Common items to avoid include

fruit drinks or cocktails, which contain more sugar than 100% fruit juice. Read food labels carefully, and watch out for code words for sugar, such as high-fructose corn sweetener, dehydrated cane juice, dextrin, dextrose, maltodextrin, sucrose, molasses, and malt syrup.

Artificial dyes and preservatives

Kids with ADHD are harmed by food additives, and those kids without can also become hyperactive from food additives such as artificial coloring and flavors, along with the preservative sodium benzoate. To prevent hyperactivity in your child, steer clear of brightly colored cereals like Fruit Loops and Lucky Charms, and choose low-sugar alternatives like Cheerios. Replace sugary drinks such as fruit punches and soft drinks with 100% fruit juice, as most of these contain artificial colors and flavors. If your child is craving a snack, consider offering them Pepperidge Farm Chessmen cookies, which are free of artificial dyes and contain lower amounts of sugar.

Foods that cause allergies

Studies have shown that some children may experience a lack of focus and increased hyperactivity due to the consumption of gluten, wheat, corn, and soy. It's been recommended that all children undergo screening for food allergies before being prescribed medication for ADHD. You discuss the possibility of allergy testing with your healthcare provider.

Nutritional supplements for ADHD

Some specialists advise individuals with ADHD to consume a daily 100% vitamin and mineral supplement. However, other nutrition experts believe that individuals who follow a normal, well-balanced diet do not require vitamins or micronutrient supplements. They assert that no scientific proof exists that such supplements assist all children with the condition.

Although multivitamins may suffice for children, adolescents, and adults who do not follow balanced diets, excessive amounts of vitamins can be harmful. It is advisable to avoid them. ADHD symptoms differ from person to person. If you're contemplating taking a supplement, it's crucial to collaborate closely with your doctor.

Healthy eating habits for impulsive, dopamine-starved ADHD brains

For adults with ADHD, maintaining healthy eating habits can be difficult. This is because studies have shown that we are required to make numerous decisions about food and eating daily, which demand strong executive functions. To establish and maintain a healthy diet, individuals with ADHD must anticipate, plan, coordinate, and execute wise food choices. The inability to meet these demands tends to demoralize people with ADHD, and they hold themselves responsible, even when their ADHD symptoms are to blame. Cultivating healthy eating habits and achieving a healthy weight starts with comprehending your ADHD brain. These are some of the most common challenges associated with developing healthy eating habits and strategies for overcoming them.

Practice mindful eating

Individuals with ADHD often struggle to be mindful of their eating habits, including what, how much, when, and where they eat. As a result, you may consume more calories than you realize and fewer healthy foods. Even if you do not enjoy your food, you might find yourself eating larger portions. Therefore, it's crucial to assess your current eating habits honestly before making any dietary changes.

- Keep a record of your food intake for a week. You can either write it down, take photos of your meals before eating them, or use notes on your phone. At the end of each day and the week, reflect on what you have consumed and compare it to your recollection. You might be surprised at the results!
- Establish specific meal times and try to eat only when hungry, not out of boredom. For instance, you could schedule breakfast at 8 a.m., a mid-morning snack at 11 a.m., lunch at 1 p.m., an afternoon snack at 3 p.m., dinner at 6 p.m., and an evening snack at 8 p.m.
- Make a habit of eating at a table instead of multitasking. People with ADHD often eat while doing other activities, like studying, watching TV, or even driving, so it's important to create a designated eating space in your home.
- Be mindful of your portion sizes, as the ADHD brain tends to crave larger volumes of food. A helpful tip is to use smaller plates and bowls, as a full bowl will still leave you feeling satisfied regardless of its size.

Curb impulsive eating

One of the defining characteristics of ADHD is impulsivity, which can manifest in eating behaviors. If you've ever eaten to the point where your stomach aches and you wonder why you did it, then you may understand this phenomenon. People with ADHD tend to eat their food quickly, which can overeat because their stomachs don't have enough time to signal to their brains that they are full. Here's how you can curb impulsive eating:

1. Drink a glass of water before a meal to help you feel satisfied sooner
2. Take a few deep breaths before eating
3. Take 20 seconds to ground yourself before eating, which can help you become a more mindful eater
4. Serve yourself a portion and give yourself time to determine whether you are truly still hungry
5. Put your fork or spoon down after each bite, and don't pick it back up until you have swallowed
6. Avoid nibbling while preparing meals, as it can lead to unintentionally consuming full meals
7. Keep snacks out of sight to avoid temptation. Seeing trigger foods can make you feel hungry and lead to impulsive snacking

Avoid emotional eating

During times of stress, it's common for everyone to turn to comfort foods like ice cream. However, adults with ADHD often struggle with emotional regulation, making them particularly prone to impulsive eating.

1. Make a list of activities to do when feeling bored rather than turning to food. Activities like calling a friend, reading a book, or doing a puzzle can be helpful distractions.
2. When feeling anxious or angry, take five minutes to breathe deeply and ground yourself. Rather than using food for sensory relief, try other soothing techniques.
3. Find creative ways to express your emotions, such as singing, movement, or martial arts. Alternatively, talk to someone about your feelings instead of impulsively turning to food.
4. Negative emotions can make you vulnerable to mindless eating, so be aware of them and take a pause before giving in to the impulse to eat.

Let the labels guide you

Navigating through the abundance of nutritional information out there can be overwhelming for adults with ADHD. Here are some simple guidelines to help take the guesswork out of healthy eating:

1. Make sure to have healthy staples on your grocery list and in your home. Having nutritious options readily available can prevent impulsive unhealthy eating. Consider stocking up on items like eggs, turkey, nuts, fish, fruits and vegetables, and boneless chicken breast.
2. Boost your meals with protein and fiber-rich foods. If you have dietary restrictions, consult a nutritionist or physician for advice on suitable alternatives.
3. Read food labels carefully to avoid underestimating the number of calories or fat in your food. When ordering takeout, check the nutritional information beforehand to make informed choices. Remember, what you don't eat can be just as influential as what you do.
4. Avoid drinking your calories. Sodas and alcoholic beverages are high in calories and can trigger impulsive behavior. Diet soda, although sugar-free, contains artificial sweeteners that may increase cravings. Choose flavored seltzer water instead, and keep in mind that juicing fruits removes fiber and increases blood sugar levels.

Hold the big picture in mind

Adults with ADHD often struggle to turn their good intentions into action. In order to achieve their goals, they need to develop healthy habits that go beyond just healthy eating.

1. Dedicate an hour each week, perhaps on the weekend, to meal planning for the coming week. Check your fridge and pantry to ensure you have all the necessary ingredients and create a shopping list for any missing items. This planning can ease decision-making during busy workdays. Put on some music, make a cup of tea, and plan ahead. Spending one hour doing this can save you the daily chore of figuring out what to eat.
2. Get enough sleep. Lack of sleep can contribute to unhealthy weight gain and worsen ADHD symptoms. When you don't get enough sleep, your body is designed to lower your metabolism and hold onto body fat as a survival mechanism. Your brain and body don't understand that you stayed up late binge-watching Netflix.
3. Exercise regularly. It can help regulate your appetite, moods, cognitive clarity, and ADHD symptoms.

PHYSICAL EXERCISE

Although medication and behavioral therapies are the standard treatments for ADHD, physical exercise is emerging as a promising complementary therapy. Exercise has been shown to improve executive function, attention, and mood, which are all areas of deficit in individuals with ADHD. In this context, physical exercise can serve as a low-risk, low-cost, and easily accessible intervention for individuals with ADHD.

How exercise affects the brain

Regular exercise has many benefits for brain health, no matter if an individual has ADHD or not. Exercise stimulates the production of various chemicals in the brain, such as neurotransmitters and growth factors, which help to support the growth of new brain cells and the formation of new neural pathways. These benefits make exercise a valuable tool for promoting mental health and well-being and may be especially beneficial for individuals with ADHD.

It can improve memory

Memory loss is a common issue that can occur as we age, and it is often linked to changes in blood flow to the brain. As we age, our large arteries and veins tend to stiffen, leading to reduced efficiency in blood circulation, including to the brain. To combat this issue and prevent memory loss, regular exercise is very effective. Both aerobic (longer duration, lower intensity) and anaerobic (shorter duration, higher intensity) exercise can improve cardiovascular function and help counter the stiffening of the vascular system.

It can enhance learning

Brain plasticity - the ability of the nervous system to change its activity in response to internal or external stimuli is a critical element in the learning process. Studies reveal that regular exercise can improve brain plasticity, allowing individuals to retain new mental and physical skills. Exercise accomplishes this by altering communication between brain cells, leading to enhanced learning and cognitive function.

It can improve mood

Regular exercise not only benefits the physical body but also has significant effects on mental health. One of the most notable effects is improving mood and overall well-being. After a high-intensity workout or a good run, you may have experienced a "runner's high," which results from a release of feel-good chemicals in the brain, such as endorphins and endocannabinoids. These substances contribute to the mood-lifting effects of exercise. Research also suggests that physical activity can significantly reduce the risk of depression. Therefore, incorporating regular exercise into your routine will not only improve your physical health but also boost your mood and prevent the development of depression.

It helps prevent or delay the onset of certain brain diseases

According to various studies, engaging in regular exercise could delay or even prevent certain brain diseases. Research has shown that physical activity is linked to a decrease in age-related cognitive decline and could delay the onset of Alzheimer's disease and other brain disorders. While the type and duration of exercise required for these benefits are not yet specified, the American Heart Association (AHA) suggests a general guideline of 150 minutes of moderate-intensity aerobic exercise per week, preferably spread throughout the week. It is also recommended to perform moderate to high-intensity strength training twice a week to maximize health benefits.

How exercise affects ADHD

Regular exercise is considered one of the most effective treatments for children and adults with Attention-Deficit/Hyperactivity Disorder (ADHD). Although exercise provides many benefits, it has unique positive effects on individuals with ADHD.

Best exercises for adults with ADHD

If you are an adult with ADHD, you might want to try a combination of aerobic and resistance training to get the most out of your exercise routine. Sure, most research interventions for adults with ADHD use aerobic exercise, but why not mix it up, right? You can try the following:

- Running
- Cycling
- Rowing
- Martial arts
- Elliptical
- Spinning
- Hiking

- Boxing
- Weightlifting

Variety is the key to avoiding getting mentally burnt out and keeping your focus in check. Since adults tend to have busier schedules, it's best to set aside time each day for exercise to stay consistent and efficient.

STRESS MANAGEMENT

If you have ADHD, managing stress is super important because your attention, focus, and impulsivity problems can make you extra vulnerable to it. You could try working out, practicing mindfulness, meditating, doing breathing exercises, or using relaxation techniques to manage stress. Just remember to work with a healthcare professional to create a personalized stress management plan that works for you. Let's delve into how you can manage stress when you have ADHD.

Managing Stress When You Have ADHD

Families dealing with ADHD symptoms often go through a lot of stress, whether it's a child or an adult with ADHD. Some adults with ADHD complain that stress always makes their ADHD symptoms worse, and when their symptoms aren't controlled, it creates more stress. Could it be that ADHD symptoms cause daily disarray that makes people feel stressed, or does stress worsen ADHD symptoms?

Well, the not-so-clear-cut answer to that is the relationship between ADHD and stress is complicated. Experts say it's likely a two-way street - ADHD symptoms can cause stress, and stress can make those symptoms even worse. This is supported by research. So, when someone says that stress is making their ADHD symptoms worse, there's quite a bit of evidence to back that up. On the other side of that, ADHD symptoms themselves can also be a source of stress.

Research into stress and ADHD symptoms

Looking into the connection between stress and ADHD, researchers have found that a majority of adults report feeling stressed out over various situations in their lives. According to the American Institute of Stress, around 73% of people experience psychological symptoms, and 77% of people report physical symptoms. Researchers also noticed that ADHD symptoms are linked to stress, particularly for adults who mainly have inattentive presentation. Chronic stress can worsen the symptoms and cause chemical and architectural changes to the brain, affecting its ability to function properly.

Another study found that stress affects the prefrontal cortex, the same area of the brain affected by ADHD. When stress hits, it reduces neuronal firing and impairs cognitive abilities. Stress can cause changes to the brain over time. It can decrease the executive functioning abilities of the brain, which can be seen in a person's ability to organize information and activities, and to manage their emotions. Stress at toxic or chronic levels can even affect brain structure and size, as well as brain function related to some of the brain chemicals.

Combined stress and ADHD symptoms can also harm personal relationships. People with ADHD and high-stress levels often have a shorter fuse and blurt out things they shouldn't say, which can lead to negative feedback and rejection. It becomes a vicious cycle where relationships get impaired, leading to more stress.

Find the middle point between being stressed and being able

To manage stress better and lessen its impact on ADHD symptoms, it's very important to tackle both the cognitive and emotional challenges when dealing with stress. There are a few techniques that can help you calm down when you're feeling stressed out, like practicing mindfulness and deep breathing. Another good way to reduce stress is to create and stick to routines and systems that can help automate your daily life and limit the number of decisions you have to make.

Once you're feeling calmer, it's a good idea to take a critical look at the situation and see if there are any ways you can improve or change it. Think about whether the problem is a poor match between what's required and your skills, especially when it comes to work. There are also other techniques that can help you manage stress, like incorporating more exercise into your routine or finding personal hobbies that help you unwind. If you're a parent, working with your partner to give yourself more alone time can also be helpful.

If stress is still getting in the way, it might be a good idea to talk to your doctor about it. They can help you come up with a treatment plan or connect you with other health professionals who can offer additional support.

The importance of managing stress

If you're feeling stressed out, it's not just your emotions that are at risk - it can seriously mess with your physical health too. Stress can make it tough to think straight, get things done, and enjoy life in general. It might seem like there's nothing you can do about it, what with everything on the go - bills piling up, endless work, and family responsibilities. The great news is you have more control than you realize.

Good stress management techniques can help you get a handle on stress and take back control of your life so that you can be happier, healthier, and more productive. The end goal is a balanced life where you have time for work, relationships, relaxation, and fun and can handle whatever challenges come your way. But everyone's different, so you might need to experiment a little to find what works best for you. Here are some tips to get you started.

Tip 1: Identify the sources of stress in your life

Managing stress starts with figuring out what's causing it in the first place. Identifying big stressors like a breakup, moving, or changing jobs might seem easy, but chronic stress is a different story. Sometimes we don't realize that our own thoughts, attitudes, and actions can be the root of our daily stress. For instance, you might be super anxious about work deadlines, but it could be your procrastination that's the real culprit.

To uncover the true sources of your stress, take a closer look at your habits, mindset, and excuses. Do you brush off stress as a temporary thing, even though you never really take a break? Do you think of stress as a normal part of life or your personality? Do you blame your stress on others or outside factors rather than looking inward? It'll be hard to get it under control until you start taking responsibility for your role in creating or maintaining stress.

A helpful way to identify sources of stress is by keeping a stress journal. A stress journal can be a useful tool to help you figure out what causes stress in your life and how you deal with it. Whenever you feel stressed, jot it down in your journal or use a stress tracker app on your phone. By keeping a daily record, you'll be able to spot patterns and recurring themes. Be sure to note down:

- What triggered your stress (even if you're not sure)
- How you felt emotionally and physically

- How you reacted to stress
- What actions you took to feel better

Tip 2: Practice the 4 A's of stress management

Stress is an automatic response from your nervous system, but some stressors arise at predictable times, like your daily commute, meetings with your boss, or family gatherings. When dealing with these kinds of predictable stressors, you can either change the situation or change your reaction. To decide which option to choose, it helps to think of the four A's: avoid, alter, adapt, or accept.

1. Avoid unnecessary stress

Don't get me wrong, sometimes you've got to face the music and deal with the stressful situations in your life. But the good news is, you can actually ditch some of those stressors that aren't really serving you. Here are a few ways to help you say goodbye to unnecessary stress:

- **Learn to say "no" and set boundaries.** This is a big one for a lot of people. It's okay to know your limits and not take on more than you can handle. Don't let people guilt you into doing things you don't want to do.
- **Avoid people who stress you out.** If there are people in your life who are bringing you down, limit your time with them or cut them off completely.

- **Take control of your surroundings.** If the news or traffic is giving you anxiety, make some changes. Turn off the TV/radio or take a different route. And if grocery shopping is a nightmare for you, just order your groceries online.
- **Look at your to-do list** and figure out what's really necessary. Drop the tasks that aren't important or delegate them to someone else. There's no need to overwhelm yourself with unnecessary tasks.

2. Alter the situation

If you can't avoid a stressful situation, try changing it up. This often involves tweaking the way you communicate and operate in your daily life.

- **Speak up and express your feelings rather than bottling them up.** If something or someone is getting under your skin, be more assertive and communicate your concerns directly and respectfully. For instance, if you're trying to study for an exam and your roommate is being chatty, let them know that you only have a few minutes to chat. Otherwise, you'll build up resentment and stress.
- **Be willing to make compromises.** If you ask someone to change their behavior, be open to doing the same. If both of you are willing to compromise a bit, you'll have a better chance of finding a happy middle ground.

- **Create a balanced schedule**. Too much work and not enough fun can lead to burnout. Aim to strike a balance between work and family life, social activities and alone time, and daily responsibilities and downtime.

3. Adapt to the stressor

If you can't change the stressor, try changing yourself. You can adapt to stressful situations and regain control by adjusting your expectations and attitude.

- **Reframe problems**. Look at stressful situations from a more positive perspective. Rather than getting angry about a traffic jam, see it as an opportunity to take a break, listen to your favorite podcast or music, or enjoy some quiet time.
- **Consider the big picture.** Take a step back and assess the situation. Ask yourself if it will matter in the end. Will it still be important in a month or a year? If not, redirect your focus and energy elsewhere.
- **Adjust your standards**. Striving for perfection often leads to unnecessary stress. Avoid setting yourself up for failure by aiming for reasonable standards for yourself and others. Be content with good enough.
- **Practice gratitude**. When stress gets to be too much, take a moment to appreciate the positive things in your life, including your own positive qualities and

talents. This simple practice can help you maintain perspective.

4. Accept the things you can't change

Some stressors are unavoidable, such as the death of a loved one, a serious illness, or a recession. In such cases, the best way to cope with stress is to practice acceptance. Although it may be challenging, it is ultimately easier than resisting a situation that cannot be changed.

- **Don't try to control the uncontrollable**. Many things in life are outside our control, especially the actions of others. Rather than worrying about them, focus on what you can control, such as your reaction to the problem.
- **Look for the silver lining**. Try to see the glass as half full. When faced with major challenges, try to view them as opportunities for personal growth. If your own mistakes contributed to a stressful situation, reflect on them, and learn from them.
- **Learn to forgive**. A wise person once said unforgiveness is like drinking poison and expecting the other person to die. These are very potent words. Recognize that we live in an imperfect world and that everyone makes mistakes. Let go of anger and resentment. Free yourself from negative energy by forgiving and moving forward.

- **Share your feelings.** Expressing what you're going through can be very therapeutic, even if you cannot change the stressful situation. Talk to a trusted friend or seek help from a therapist.

Tip 3: Get moving

Exercising may be the last thing you want to do when you're stressed, but it's a great way to relieve stress; you don't need to be an athlete or spend hours in a gym to reap the benefits. Physical activity releases endorphins that boost your mood, and it can also distract you from daily worries.

While regular exercise for 30 minutes or more is ideal, you can start small and gradually increase your fitness level. Every little bit helps. The first step is to get moving. You can incorporate exercise into your daily routine by

- Turning on some music and dancing
- Taking your dog for a walk
- Cycling or walking to the store
- Using stairs instead of elevators at home or work
- Parking your car far away and walking the rest of the distance
- Finding an exercise partner and encouraging each other
- Playing a game, like ping-pong or active video games with your kids

You can also blow off some steam by trying out mindful rhythmic exercises with stress-busting magic, like walking, running, swimming, dancing, cycling, tai chi, and aerobics, which can really help you get into a better headspace. The key is to pick something you enjoy doing, so you're more likely to stick with it.

When you're working out, try to focus on your body and how it feels. Pay attention to your breathing and how it coordinates with your movements or notice how the sun feels on your skin. By being more mindful during your exercise routine, you'll be able to break free from those negative thoughts that tend to weigh you down when you're stressed.

Tip 4: Connect to others

Hanging out with your favorite people is one of the most soothing things you can do when you're stressed. There's something about being around people who understand you and make you feel comfortable that triggers a release of hormones that counter your body's stress response. It's like a natural remedy for stress, and it has the added benefit of fighting off anxiety and depression. Make every effort to connect with family and friends on a regular basis, in person if possible.

Remember, your friends and family don't have to fix your problems. They just need to listen without judgment. Don't let the fear of being vulnerable or a burden stop you from opening. Your loved ones will appreciate your trust and it will only strengthen your relationship. Of course, it's not always easy to have someone close by to turn to when stress hits, but by building and maintaining a supportive network of close friends, you'll be better equipped to handle life's challenges.

You can cultivate relationships and connect with others in these ways:

- Talk to a coworker during a break
- Volunteer to help someone else
- Have lunch or coffee with a friend
- Ask a loved one to check in with you regularly
- Go to a movie or attend a concert with someone
- Call or email an old friend
- Go for a walk with a workout buddy
- Schedule a weekly dinner date with someone
- Join a club or take a class to meet new people
- Confide in a teacher, sports coach, or clergy member

Tip 5: Make time for fun and relaxation

To help lower your stress levels, it's important to have some 'me' time and have some fun. You don't want to get so caught up in everything else that you forget to look after yourself! Taking time to relax and have fun is essential, not just a luxury. Here are some ways to help you carve out that much-needed 'me' time:

- **Schedule leisure time daily**. This is your chance to take a break from your responsibilities and recharge your batteries.
- **Do something you enjoy daily**. Whether it's playing an instrument, staring up at the stars, or tinkering with your bike, make sure to take some time to do what you love.
- **Don't forget to keep a sense of humor!** Laughing, even at yourself, can help your body fight stress in many ways. As they say, laughter is the best medicine.
- **Try out a relaxation practice** like yoga, meditation, or deep breathing. These techniques can help activate your body's relaxation response, the opposite of the fight-flight response. With practice, you'll be able to lower your stress levels and find some calm and centering.

Tip 6: Manage your time better

Bad time management can add to the stress. When you're trying to do too many things at once and falling behind, it can leave you feeling pretty frazzled. And when you're stressed out like that, it's easy to let go of all the healthy habits you know you should be doing, like hanging out with friends and getting enough sleep. But don't worry, there are some things you can do to balance your work and personal life better.

- **Don't over-commit yourself.** Don't try to do too many things in one day or back-to-back. It's easy to think you can do it all, but you'll probably end up underestimating how long things take and stressing yourself out even more.
- **Make a list of everything you need to do and prioritize them.** Start with the most important tasks and tackle them first. If there's something particularly unpleasant on the list, get it done early on so you can enjoy the rest of your day.
- **Break down tasks and projects into bite size, manageable steps.** Focus on one step at a time rather than trying to take on everything at once.
- **Don't be afraid to delegate tasks** to other people. You don't have to do everything yourself, whether it's at work or at home. If someone else can handle it, let them. It'll take some of the pressure off you and help you avoid unnecessary stress.

Tip 7: Maintain balance with a healthy lifestyle

Besides working out, you can make some healthy lifestyle choices that'll help you feel more resilient too.

- **Eat healthy.** It will give your body the fuel it needs to handle stress. Try to eat balanced, nutritious meals throughout the day, and don't skip breakfast.

- **Reduce caffeine and sugar**. They can give you a quick burst of energy, but then you'll crash and feel even worse.
- **Avoid alcohol, cigarettes, and drugs** when you're feeling stressed. Using these to escape may seem like a quick fix, but it won't solve anything in the end. Instead, try to face your problems head-on with a clear mind.
- **Get enough sleep.** Being tired can make you feel even more stressed out and cause you to think irrationally. So, try to get some good quality sleep each night to help you feel refreshed and ready to take on whatever comes your way in the day.

Tip 8: Learn to relieve stress in the moment

Life can get overwhelming sometimes. Whether you're dealing with a frustrating commute, a tough day at work, or a disagreement with your significant other, you need some quick and easy ways to manage your stress levels. That's where quick stress relief techniques come in handy. The easiest way to reduce stress fast is by taking a deep breath and using your senses. You can try looking at a favorite photo, smelling a calming scent, listening to a favorite song, tasting a piece of candy, or snuggling with a pet. Everyone's different, so it's important to experiment and find out which sensory experiences work best for you.

The important thing is to find what works for you and make it a go-to when you're feeling frazzled. With a little practice, you'll be able to quickly calm yourself down and tackle whatever challenges come your way.

MINDFULNESS AND ADHD

Medication and therapy aren't your only options for managing ADHD symptoms. Recent research suggests that mindfulness meditation, which involves actively observing your thoughts and feelings in the present moment, can be a helpful tool for calming your mind and improving your focus. According to a survey, over a third of adults with ADHD practice mindfulness meditation, with around 40% giving it high ratings. The great thing about mindfulness meditation is that you don't need a prescription or a therapist's office to practice it. You can do it anywhere, whether sitting or walking. It's a convenient and accessible option for those seeking other ways to manage their ADHD symptoms.

Mindfulness is the practice of paying focused attention to your thoughts, feelings, and bodily sensations, which helps to develop a deeper awareness of your current state in the moment. This technique can be used as a powerful tool to promote overall wellness, particularly when it comes to psychological well-being. In fact, similar techniques have been used to alleviate stress and mood disorders.

How it works

Mindfulness meditation can enhance your capacity to regulate attention, enabling you to develop the skill of self-observation and the ability to concentrate on a specific task. This technique also helps to train your mind to refocus on the present moment when it wanders, and to heighten your awareness of your emotions, which reduces impulsive reactions. Research suggests that mindfulness meditation may benefit those with ADHD by increasing the thickness of the pre-frontal cortex, a region of the brain responsible for focus, planning, and impulse control. Additionally, this technique can raise levels of dopamine in the brain, which is typically lower in individuals with ADHD.

A significant study revealed that individuals with ADHD who participated in a weekly 2.5-hour mindfulness meditation session, coupled with a daily home practice that gradually increased from 5 to 15 minutes over 8 weeks, experienced enhanced focus, and concentration on tasks. These individuals reported decreased levels of anxiety and depression. Other studies have since produced comparable findings, further substantiating the positive impact of mindfulness meditation on individuals with ADHD.

Practicing mindfulness on your own

The basic practice of mindfulness meditation is straightforward. Simply find a comfortable place to sit where you won't be disturbed and spend five minutes focusing on your breath. Notice the sensation of breathing in and breathing out, monitoring the rising and falling of your stomach. You may soon find that your mind starts to wander, perhaps to thoughts about work, outside noises, or plans for later in the day. When this happens, simply label those thoughts as thinking, and return your focus to your breath. The mind is naturally prone to distraction, and the practice of mindful awareness is not about staying fixed on the breath, but about consistently redirecting your attention back to the breath. This process of repeatedly shifting your focus is what strengthens your ability to concentrate. For individuals with ADHD, this emphasis on refocusing attention can be particularly beneficial, as it helps to counter the mind's innate tendency to wander.

It's important to make this a daily habit, gradually increasing the time you spend every couple of weeks. You can also incorporate mindfulness into your everyday activities, such as focusing on your breath for a few minutes while taking a walk or sitting at your desk, or even during conversations with others. The goal is to cultivate a mind-awareness state throughout your day, letting go of the busyness of your thoughts and bringing your attention to what's happening in the present moment. With practice, mindfulness can become a valuable tool for improving focus and reducing stress in everyday life.

SUMMARY

- People with ADHD are more likely to experience sleep-related issues
- Getting enough sleep can improve the quality of life of individuals with ADHD
- Common sleep disorders that people with ADHD might experience include insomnia, circadian rhythm sleep disorders, narcolepsy, and restless leg syndrome among others
- Practicing good sleep hygiene can improve sleep, ADHD symptoms, daily functioning, and behavior
- Eating nutritious food high in protein, complex carbohydrates, and omega-3 fatty acids can positively impact the functionality of your brain
- Avoid foods that are high in sugar, artificial dyes and preservatives, and allergy-causing foods
- Physical exercise is a promising complementary therapy for ADHD
- A combination of aerobic and resistance training exercises is recommended
- Stress management is especially important for people with ADHD because your attention, focus, and impulsivity problems can make you extra vulnerable to it
- Practicing mindfulness and deep breathing can help in managing stress

- Good stress management techniques can help you get a handle on stress
- Practicing mindfulness is a great way to manage ADHD symptoms

Now you know how important good health, exercise, and stress management are, let's turn our focus to managing emotions and rejection sensitivity in the next chapter.

4

MANAGING EMOTIONS & REJECTION SENSITIVITY

A DECADE LOST

I read a really touching story about a woman who lost a decade of her life due to medical negligence. She had symptoms of ADHD, but they were dismissed by her psychiatrist, who diagnosed her with depression and anxiety instead. How disappointing! The perception of ADHD as a disorder that affects only boys and men has resulted in girls and women with ADHD being underdiagnosed or misdiagnosed. This woman suffered from social isolation, emotional manipulation, gaslighting, comorbid mood disorders, rejection sensitive dysphoria, and self-harm.

Commonly prescribed antidepressants, such as selective serotonin reuptake inhibitors (SSRIs), only worsened her symptoms. The woman struggled through college, and her career suffered as she could not show her talent due to her symptoms. After trying *multiple medications and treatments, she was diagnosed with Bipolar II. She was then eventually diagnosed with ADHD a decade later! Unbelievable!*

Reading this woman's story made me wanna cry with indignation. No one should have to go through what she went through - confusion, helplessness, and hopelessness. It must suck to know what you know and doctors make it seem like you're crazy for even thinking it. My heart goes out to all the women suffering through misdiagnoses, apathy, and egotism from medical professionals. I think doctors need to start listening to their patients and taking their symptoms seriously to avoid dangerous medical negligence.

EXAGGERATED EMOTIONS

For people with ADHD, trouble processing emotions starts with the brain, which can lead to emotional dysregulation. Around 70% of adults with ADHD experience emotional regulation challenges. ADHD and emotional dysregulation are closely intertwined since the way the ADHD brain is wired makes it difficult to regulate emotions. Let's look at how ADHD can cause emotional dysregulation.

Emotions rule

Most doctors don't really think about emotional challenges when giving an ADHD diagnosis. The DSM-5 - Diagnostic and Statistical Manual of Mental Disorders, 5th edition, doesn't include emotional dysregulation as part of the diagnostic criteria for ADHD. But recent research has shown that people with ADHD have a harder time dealing with low frustration tolerance, impatience, temper, and excitability compared to people without ADHD.

Processing emotion: a brain thing

Dealing with emotions can be a struggle for people with ADHD, as it often begins in the brain. Because of issues with their working memory, a tiny feeling can blow up into something big that takes over their mind. On top of that, some people with ADHD may seem indifferent or unaware of other people's emotions. The brain connectivity networks responsible for processing emotions seem somewhat restricted in individuals with ADHD.

Fastening on a feeling

When a teenager with ADHD, for example, gets angry when a parent denies them the use of the car, this exaggerated emotional response may be due to 'flooding.' This means that a momentary emotion can become so overpowering that it takes up all the space in the mind, like a computer bug that takes up all the space on a hard drive. Consequently, the teen cannot focus on other relevant information that could help them manage their anger and control their actions.

Extreme sensitivity to disapproval

People with ADHD can often get caught up in one intense emotion and struggle to shift their focus to other aspects of a situation. For example, they may perceive a coworker's response as critical after hearing just a hint of uncertainty and react defensively without fully listening to the coworker's input. This difficulty in emotional regulation can cause inappropriate outbursts that may damage relationships and hinder productivity in the workplace.

Bottled up by fear

More than one-third of teens and adults with ADHD experience significant social anxiety as a chronic problem. They often live with persistent fears of being perceived by others as inadequate, unattractive, or uncool.

Giving in to avoidance and denial

Some individuals with ADHD struggle with managing important emotions effectively. They may have trouble tolerating strong emotions and resort to certain behaviors to avoid feeling overwhelmed. For instance, they may avoid meeting new people or postpone important tasks to avoid anxiety or stress.

Carried away with emotion

Many individuals with ADHD struggle to regulate their emotions because their brain's gating mechanism does not differentiate between major threats and minor issues. This means they might feel stressed or panicked over things that are non-threatening, which makes it harder for them to handle stressful situations logically.

Sadness and low self-esteem

People with untreated ADHD can experience dysthymia, a long-term and mild mood disorder characterized by persistent sadness. This condition can arise from living with challenges, disappointments, negative feedback, and life stress resulting from untreated or inadequately treated ADHD. Those who have dysthymia may experience low energy and self-esteem daily.

Emotions and getting started

People with untreated ADHD may find it hard to get motivated for tasks that offer long-term rewards. Instead, they tend to focus on activities that provide immediate satisfaction. As a result, they may struggle to initiate and maintain the effort for tasks that require delayed gratification.

Emotions and getting started 2

Brain imaging studies reveal that individuals with ADHD have fewer receptor sites for chemicals that activate reward-recognizing circuits in the brain compared to those without ADHD. This means that people with ADHD have trouble anticipating pleasure or experiencing satisfaction with tasks that offer delayed rewards.

Emotions and working memory

When working memory, your feelings play a big role, whether you realize it or not, giving you the boost, you need to get organized, concentrate, keep track of things, and keep your behavior in check. Many individuals with ADHD have an inadequate working memory, which may explain why they are often disorganized, quick-tempered, or procrastinate.

EMOTIONAL REGULATION AND REDIRECTION

Being able to control and channel emotions in a positive way is key to emotional regulation and redirection. It means recognizing and making sense of your feelings, managing how you react to them, and dealing with things that set them off. Learning how to do this can be a big help for people with ADHD in managing their symptoms and feeling better overall.

Emotional regulation challenges

Have you ever hesitated to commit to a future appointment, arrangement, or task? Do you worry that you may not be in the right headspace to tackle the task at that future time? This is often dismissed as avoidance, procrastination, or an unwillingness to commit. However, ADHD often leads to emotional regulation and redirection challenges, which can result in heightened emotional reactivity and difficulty in engaging with others. These emotional experiences can feel out of control and lead to problems with time projection and motivation. Adults with ADHD struggle with managing their emotions, which makes it harder for them to pay attention and stay on track. It can be tough for them to handle their feelings in a way that helps them focus and look at things in a positive light.

The two stages of emotion

Sometimes you can't control your emotions and react without thinking. This happens because your brain struggles to regulate emotions, especially when you're processing new information. Depending on past experiences, you may feel excited, turned off, or disinterested. Ideally, your brain would activate the Task Positive Network (TPN) to focus on details and plan actions. Simultaneously, the default mode network (DMN) takes a back seat, which can change how you feel. This helps you control your emotions and choose how to act. But people with ADHD might struggle with this because their brain doesn't activate the right networks. Sometimes, their TPN doesn't activate as it should, and their DMN doesn't quiet down enough. This makes it tough to control their feelings or choose how to act, but on the bright side, they can still work to change their behavior.

What we can change

To stop being so reactive to your emotions and take charge of how you feel, there are some things you can do to get there. First, you need to activate your attention. That means creating an emotional reference point and practicing inhibition. You can think of it as priming, pausing, and projecting.

Priming means setting up a stable emotional foundation for yourself. There are two ways to do this: general and specific.

For general positive emotional priming, imagine how you want to feel and react to challenges throughout the day. Create a mental picture of yourself feeling positive and in control, and plan when to revisit this image throughout the day. Specific positive emotional priming is preparing for a specific situation by imagining yourself as the best version of yourself.

Pausing. When feeling emotional, the pause button can help you regain control. You could try taking deep breaths, counting slowly from ten, or just walking away for a moment. If you have ADHD, this can be extra hard because emotions can be intense, and it can be tough to stop yourself from acting impulsively. One thing that can help is paying attention to physical signals that you're starting to feel overwhelmed, like feeling hot or having trouble breathing. If you notice these signs, try taking a pause before things get too intense.

Projecting means directing your attention and emotions toward a specific goal. To feel a specific emotion, you need to focus your attention on it. It's not as hard as it sounds. Start by reinforcing your ability to choose your emotional response. Imagine doing something you want to do and focusing on all the positives. If negative thoughts pop up, acknowledge them but then focus on creating a mental solution and replace the negative thoughts with positive ones.

1. **Reinforce your ability to choose** by thinking of a future activity and asking yourself, "How will I choose to feel when that day or moment comes?"
2. **Build a mental image** by imagining all the positives related to that activity. Visualize yourself going through the motions of doing it and enjoying the benefits. Take note of how you're dressed, how the interactions will go, and what you'll gain from it.
3. **Defuse any negative thoughts** that come up by acknowledging them and reminding yourself that you have the power to choose how you feel. Then create a mental solution and replace the negative thoughts with a positive mental image.

SOLVE: a helpful tool for emotional redirection

SOLVE is a tool that adults with ADHD can use to manage their emotions when they are deep in thought. It's particularly helpful for breaking out from emotional cycles. Let's look at how to SOLVE the emotional loop.

Stop: Intentionally interrupt the emotional loop by physically changing your perspective and taking a deep calming breath.

Objective List: List only the information you know about the issue, not emotionally driven assumptions and fears. This will activate your attention to detail and highlight any knowledge gaps.

Verbalize: Speak the solution you have arrived at in simple, direct terms. If an action is needed, state when and how it will be taken.

Exit: Move on to your next task or activity, resetting your focus and attention.

Repeat: Emotionally driven thoughts may resurface, but repeating the SOLVE steps will help reduce their impact over time.

Remember that emotions are initially reactions and assigning meaning to them is up to us. By intentionally focusing on details, we can shape our emotional experience. It may require practice and utilizing tools like the SOLVE acronym, but doing so can enhance our emotional regulation and help us create experiences that benefit us.

REJECTION SENSITIVITY

As a person with ADHD, I'm sure you understand the pain that comes with rejection all too well. People with ADHD can sometimes struggle with failed relationships and difficulty managing emotions, leading to reluctance to pursue new friendships or romantic relationships. The fear of being rejected is simply too great to risk trying again. This fear of rejection, sometimes associated with ADHD, has been named rejection sensitive dysphoria (RSD). It is an aspect of adult ADHD that is often overlooked.

Individuals with ADHD may experience rejection sensitive dysphoria, which can result in heightened emotional sensitivity and intense emotional distress. This condition can mimic mood disorders and may involve suicidal thoughts or sudden bursts of rage directed towards those who caused the pain. RSD can cause a sudden shift from a stable emotional state to intense sadness, which can be misdiagnosed as a rapid cycling mood disorder.

Rejection sensitive dysphoria: a hidden condition

Rejection sensitive dysphoria is a unique emotional condition that appears to be exclusively associated with ADHD. It's when you feel sensitive and hurt when you think someone important in your life is rejecting you, criticizing you, teasing you, or that you're disappointing yourself and others. Even if it's not real, just the idea of it can be hurtful.

This kind of emotional pain is intense and hard to put into words, and because of that, people with RSD might either try hard to please others all the time or they might give up on their own goals because they're too scared to fail. They might avoid going on dates, applying for jobs, or speaking up in meetings because they fear rejection. It's important to know that this is real and not something to be dismissed. If you or someone you know is experiencing this, talking to a professional who can help you manage it might be helpful.

Coping with painful emotions

Rejection sensitivity can lead to a harmful cycle of repeating past trauma. To break this cycle, you must respond thoughtfully after considering the situation and the other person's actions rather than reacting impulsively.

You can handle rejection sensitivity using these strategies:

- Process emotions before having a meltdown by accepting and acknowledging emotions, letting go of guilt, and moving away from perfectionism
- Seek a proper diagnosis and collaborate with medical professionals to develop a treatment plan
- Going to therapy with a specialized counselor who can help develop coping strategies for strong emotions is also recommended
- Try to reduce overall stress

What you can do to manage rejection sensitivity

Rejection sensitivity is a neurological and genetic component of ADHD that may be exacerbated by early childhood trauma, but it is not solely caused by it. Many patients find comfort in simply having a name for this feeling and knowing they are not alone in their experience. It can be reassuring to learn that almost all individuals with ADHD experience rejection sensitivity. Upon receiving this diagnosis, many patients experience a sense of relief, realizing that their struggles are not their own and that they are not inherently damaged. Many people who experience rejection sensitivity often feel ashamed and may hesitate to seek help. Yet help is available, and talking to a mental health professional can be beneficial. Therapy can be valuable, particularly when it focuses on recognizing emotions and developing coping mechanisms.

Certain medications have been found to be helpful for some individuals. Pursuing effective treatment for ADHD and any coexisting conditions can also aid in managing rejection sensitivity.

WHAT ABOUT EMPATHY?

Empathy is the experience of understanding another person's condition from their perspective, which is crucial because empathy plays a significant role in human interactions. In essence, empathy involves feeling what another person is feeling rather than simply listening to or hearing about their experiences. This is something that we all crave in our lives. It's not enough to just be heard; we all want and need to be understood. When someone empathizes with us, it helps us feel seen and validated, which can be incredibly powerful and healing.

While it may be easier to experience empathy, expressing it accurately can be challenging. In that sense, empathy can be a double-edged sword for people with ADHD. Sometimes trying to empathize and be empathetic can backfire because it might not come across that way to others. For example, one woman with ADHD recounts a situation where her friend went through a breakup, and she wanted to support her. While trying to empathize with her friend, she started talking about her own past heartbreaks and unintentionally hijacked the conversation. She realized that neurotypical people might not experience emotions as intensely or hold onto them for as long, and she saw the need to be more mindful in future conversations.

Can ADHD affect empathy?

Empathy is central to emotional intelligence (EQ), the ability to recognize, understand, and hold space for your and others' emotions. But some habits, behaviors, or personality traits can create an impression of reduced empathy, even if you have high levels of it. ADHD symptoms such as restlessness, impulsivity, and difficulty focusing might suggest a lack of empathy. Additionally, individuals with ADHD may interrupt others often, get distracted easily, or react before considering their response, leading to words or actions that seem less empathetic. Many people with ADHD are highly empathetic, despite these traits. There is much to consider regarding the link between ADHD and empathy.

What does it mean to have low empathy

Having some background knowledge of how empathy differs from related responses like sympathy and compassion can help better understand empathy and how it might show up.

- Sympathy is an emotional reaction to someone's pain and distress, such as pity or sorrow. It involves feeling for them.
- Empathy, on the other hand, is the ability to acknowledge and understand someone's emotions. When you empathize with someone, you feel with them;
- Compassion involves understanding someone else's pain and having the desire to alleviate their distress in some way. It encompasses feeling for someone and taking action to help them.

Experts believe that empathy is a trait you're born with and a skill you can develop. They have also identified two distinct types of empathy: cognitive empathy and affective empathy.

Cognitive vs. affective empathy

Cognitive empathy is when you can somewhat understand what someone else is feeling just by picking up on cues like their tone of voice, facial expressions, or body language. It's like you have a basic understanding of their emotions. On the other hand, affective empathy (also called emotional empathy) is when you can really share in someone else's emotional experiences and feel with them. This kind of empathy can make you more likely to practice acts of kindness and compassion.

But some people just have less empathy than others. If that's the case for you, you might find it harder to consider other people's perspectives, forgive mistakes, or understand how other people feel. You might even be a bit critical of others or act impulsively without thinking about how it might affect them.

But don't worry, having less empathy doesn't mean you're a bad person. It's just something that varies from person to person. And the good news is that you can always work on developing your empathy skills. And if you're wondering how to show empathy, it's really just about understanding someone else's feelings and putting yourself in their shoes. So, for example, if you interrupt a friend a lot and then feel bad about it later, you might think to yourself, "Wow, I bet that's really frustrating for her when I interrupt her. I should work on that." See? Empathy in action!

Does ADHD cause low empathy?

For many individuals with ADHD, the world can seem tumultuous, daunting, and challenging to navigate. The symptoms of impulsivity and difficulty concentrating can make it difficult to comprehend and manage one's emotions, let alone understand and empathize with others. People with ADHD can sometimes find themselves in situations where they inadvertently say or do something that comes across as impolite or inappropriate.

However, this doesn't imply that people with ADHD necessarily have low empathy. Although they may occasionally get caught up in the moment and forget important details, such as meeting a friend for lunch, they often experience profound feelings of guilt and remorse when they realize their mistake and worry that they may have disappointed their friend.

How to cope

If you struggle to connect with others, it can sometimes cause problems in your relationships. But there are ways to work on it and build stronger bonds with your friends.

- Explain how your ADHD symptoms can show up. Talk about how you don't mean to hijack a conversation and cut someone off. Or you could let them know that you struggle to remember things people tell you, but you're good with written plans.
- It's also important to listen to others and monitor body language. If someone seems bored or distracted, try changing the subject or asking them a question to get their perspective.
- Don't be afraid to share your needs, either. If you tend to run late, tell your friends and family to give you a heads-up to come earlier than the planned time.

- Try getting vulnerable by sharing your own thoughts and feelings.

The spotlight effect is real. People probably don't notice your perceived flaws as much as you think they do. So even if you do slip up sometimes, it doesn't mean you're a bad person. Keep working on those communication skills and building those connections.

How therapy can help

Therapy can be a real game-changer. It can help you understand how your specific symptoms show up and how they affect your life and relationships. Without treatment, ADHD can seriously mess with your life. But a good therapist can help you:

- Figure out which symptoms are causing the most trouble for you
- Learn better ways to manage those symptoms
- Work on your communication skills so you can express your needs better
- Come up with ideas for connecting with others in more meaningful ways
- Deal with any worries you have about lacking empathy

One therapist compares therapy to going to the gym. Sure, you can work out by yourself, but to see results, a trainer can help you figure out which exercises to do and how often to do them. Similarly, if, for example, you're always running late, your therapist might help you figure out why that happens and how you can stay on schedule. Maybe you get distracted by stuff around the house, so you could work on staying focused.

Where does high empathy fit in?

Being hypersensitive is a common trait in people with ADHD. Specifically, you may struggle to filter sensory input from your environment or others, including emotional cues like changes in tone of voice or facial expressions. While some experts believe this heightened sensitivity can lead to greater empathy, it can also be overwhelming in stimulating social situations.

Here are some signs that you may be hypersensitive:

- You feel strongly affected by others' emotions and moods and struggle in situations where others express strong emotions
- You feel detached when others show intense emotional reactions
- You try to avoid overly emotional situations
- You have difficulty setting boundaries when people share intense emotions
- You withdraw from others to protect yourself
- You find it challenging to control your emotions when you feel overwhelmed

If you're struggling with hypersensitivity, try the following:

- Journaling about your emotions
- Practicing mindfulness techniques to help you manage emotional discomfort effectively
- Learning to set boundaries in relationships to protect yourself emotionally and preserve your energy
- Using exercise, deep breathing, or meditation to ease stress in emotionally charged situations

THE POWER OF GRATITUDE

Being grateful can make a big difference for people with ADHD. It helps you think more positively and feel better overall. When you focus on being thankful, you're less likely to get bogged down by negative thoughts and feelings that make it harder to concentrate. Expressing gratitude can help you connect better with others and communicate more effectively.

A magic tool for ADHD brains

The human brain is designed to prioritize survival and reproduction, which it accomplishes effectively. It also keeps us safe, supports our social connections, and effectively identifies problems that need addressing.

Why is gratitude so powerful?

Our brains are wired to constantly scan our surroundings for potential threats and dangers; not just physical harm but anything that could harm our relationships, which are crucial to our survival. Yet if we get caught up in dwelling on our mistakes, worrying about potential problems, and trying to fix everything wrong in the world, our brains can become overwhelmed with negativity, leaving us feeling pretty miserable.

That's where gratitude comes in. By focusing on the good things in our lives, we can train our brains to shift away from negativity and towards positivity. This can have a transformative effect on both our mental and physical well-being.

The impact of gratitude

Practicing gratitude can greatly impact your overall well-being - from your mental outlook to your physical health. Studies have shown that gratitude can:

- Boost your happiness levels
- Help you experience more positive emotions
- Enhance your ability to savor positive experiences
- Improve your physical health
- Enable you to better cope with challenges
- Strengthen your relationships
- Increase your productivity

- Lower your stress and anxiety levels
- Combat depression
- Ease physical pain
- Improve the quality of your sleep

Does gratitude really change the brain?

I know it might sound too good to be true, but the research doesn't lie. When you show gratitude or receive it, your brain releases dopamine and serotonin. That means you'll feel better right away. The more you practice gratitude, the better it gets. Your brain will start building new neural pathways to keep those feel-good chemicals flowing. Fancy brain scans (fMRI studies) have even shown that practicing gratitude regularly can change the way your brain is wired. It can help with your mood, decision-making skills, and even your immune system. Just what the doctor ordered!

Why is gratitude especially powerful for ADHD brains?

For a few reasons, gratitude can be powerful, especially for the ADHD brain. Let's explore these reasons.

1. Gratitude helps regulate the executive functioning system

ADHD is caused by insufficient dopamine in the prefrontal cortex, the area responsible for executive functions. Expressing or receiving gratitude can activate dopamine and serotonin release in the brain. Repeatedly practicing gratitude can strengthen the brain's pathways to efficiently utilize these neurotransmitters, resulting in positive changes and better regulation of dopamine levels. This is beneficial for individuals with ADHD who require additional support in managing their dopamine levels.

2. Gratitude reduces rejection sensitivity

People with ADHD have brains that are extra sensitive to rejection. Because of this, they tend to be on high alert, looking out for any potential rejection that may come their way. Unfortunately, this constant vigilance often backfires, causing them to experience rejection more frequently.

However, when people with ADHD practice gratitude, it shifts their focus away from the things and people that might reject them and toward all the positive things in their life. This shift in focus can actually make them feel better and protect their nervous system. Ultimately, gratitude helps people with ADHD feel safer and more secure in the world.

3. Gratitude increases productivity

Focusing on the positive aspects of our world and creating a success spiral can lead to a cycle of achievement, where we can relish our accomplishments and be motivated to continue being productive. This, in turn, sets the stage for further success and a more gratifying journey toward our goals.

4. It reduces anxiety

Our brains are unable to concentrate on both positive and negative information concurrently. Therefore, when we cultivate gratitude, we deactivate the negative loops that have developed over time and activate positive, dopamine-driven mechanisms instead. With continued practice, the focus on gratitude decreases the activation of anxiety and fear-based neural networks while strengthening new, positive ones. This leads to the gradual disintegration of the old, negative networks and the bolstering of the new, positive ones.

5. It increases resilience

Living with an ADHD brain in a neurotypical world can result in numerous mistakes, blunders, and disruptions. However, the emotional reaction to these errors can throw you off balance. Practicing gratitude regularly can mitigate the emotional turmoil caused by these failures, allowing you to concentrate on solutions and maintain a balanced sense of yourself and your life.

Gratitude exercises

There are countless ways to inject positivity into your life. The trick is to find a strategy that suits you, your life, and your brain. Here are a few ideas to get you started:

1. **Gratitude journal** - One awesome way to accumulate positivity is by keeping a gratitude

journal. Jot down 3-5 things you're grateful for each night. It's a fantastic way to gather all the positivity and have something genuinely uplifting to read through during tough times.
2. **Gratitude text buddy** - Start a buddy system with a friend to text each other 3 things you're grateful for every day. Partnering like this can help keep you accountable and on track with your gratitude practice.
3. **Gratitude social media challenge** - Get a group of friends to join you in a gratitude challenge. Post something you're grateful for each day for an entire month and encourage your friends to do the same. Seeing their posts can serve as a reminder to practice gratitude, and you might be surprised at how much better you feel by the end of that month!
4. **Family bedtime gratitude ritual** - Consider making a habit of sharing three things you're thankful for with your family every night at bedtime and encourage them to do the same. Studies suggest that although children may not experience the same mood-enhancing benefits of gratitude as adults, introducing this practice at an early age can foster greater optimism. Besides, kids can be pretty good accountability partners.
5. **Partner gratitude rituals** - Make a habit of sharing 3 things you're grateful for with your partner each evening during dinner or at bedtime. This is a

beautiful way to connect with the people you care about while sharing about your day.
6. **Gratitude meditation** - Guided gratitude meditations provide a fantastic chance to contemplate all the positive aspects of your life and help you become more aware of them throughout the rest of your day.
7. **Gratitude letters** - Write a letter to those you appreciate, expressing your gratitude for what they have done for you and explaining the reasons behind your appreciation.
8. **Gratitude lists** - Maintain a continuous record of things that you are grateful for on your phone or in a journal. This is a simple and convenient way to quickly access a dose of optimism whenever you need it.

Making gratitude work for the ADHD brain

You might be thinking, "I would love to be more grateful, but I struggle with maintaining regular practices due to my ADHD brain." Regular practice can be difficult for those with ADHD. However, remember that even one switch to gratitude can have a significant positive impact on your mood and help stop negative spirals. To make regular practice possible, we need to break it down into three key elements:

1. A plan

When developing a plan, consider the following:

- What exactly are you going to do?
- When will you do it?
- What daily activity can you tie it to? (e.g., dinner, dishes, bedtime, morning coffee)
- Where will you do it?
- What do you need to do it?

2. A cue

Next, you need cues to remind you to practice gratitude. Ideally, have both a time-based and location-based reminder. For time-based reminders, consider setting alarms. For location-based reminders, use sticky notes or place your gratitude journal in a visible location.

3. Accountability

Accountability is key. Partnering with a friend, partner, or family member can help keep you on track and maintain momentum, even on days when you don't feel like practicing gratitude.

Remember, changing your focus to the good can bring healing, light, and joy to your life. Try it by creating a pattern and setting up a routine.

SUMMARY

- ADHD can lead to emotional dysregulation
- People with ADHD have a harder time dealing with emotional situations than those without
- People with ADHD can often fixate on one intense emotion
- Some individuals with ADHD struggle with managing important emotions effectively.
- Empathy can be a double-edged sword for people with ADHD
- Therapy helps in understanding how specific symptoms show up and how they affect a person's life and relationships
- Gratitude can have a huge positive effect on your overall well-being

Managing emotions and rejection sensitivity can have a significant impact on many areas of your life, including your relationship with money. This is a perfect segue for us to focus on improving your relationship with money.

5

IMPROVING YOUR RELATIONSHIP WITH MONEY

I chatted with my therapist recently after splurging on some stuff. I didn't plan it; it kinda just happened. She explained that people with ADHD tend to prefer immediate rewards rather than waiting for a bigger reward later on. She said it's also possible to experience negative consequences throughout life, such as struggling in school, having trouble with employment, and engaging in risky behaviors like substance abuse and self-harm. Even with treatment, these difficulties can still occur. Adults with ADHD also often struggle with managing finances, including paying bills on time and using credit cards impulsively (so me!). They may rely more on family members and high-interest borrowing options like pawnshops and payday loans.

She also shared some research findings, which showed that people with ADHD tend to want more credit than the average person before they hit 30. But as they get older, their desire for credit keeps *going up while everyone else's goes down. This is because banks and lenders often say no to their credit applications, which means they can't get it even though they want it. And even when they ask for more credit, until they hit around 50, people with ADHD are usually given less new consumer credit than others. One of the reasons for this limited credit access is that folks with ADHD don't always do a great job paying their debts back. They're more likely to have new arrears than people who don't have ADHD.*

She said people with ADHD are more likely to take their own lives than people without. And it's not just a problem when they're young; it's pretty much a risk at any age up to 60. The difference in suicide rates between people with and without ADHD is actually pretty huge. And when you add in financial troubles, things can get even worse. People with ADHD with poor credit are at even higher risk for suicide.

Wow, I did not know that! My therapist has advised that I evaluate my relationship with money. With all these hard-hitting facts, she's not far off the mark.

IT'S HARDER TO MANAGE FINANCES

People with ADHD may struggle to manage their finances and have a higher propensity for getting into debt and fighting about money with their significant other because of attention and impulse control difficulties, leading to impulsive purchases and forgetfulness about bills. The ability to plan and organize finances may also be impacted by ADHD symptoms such as procrastination and difficulty with decision-making. These challenges can lead to financial stress and difficulties with debt management.

Let's zoom in and see what that looks like.

A pattern of financial behavior

Some common traits in adults with ADHD when it comes to money include:

- **Living paycheck to paycheck** - ADHD can often come with a lack of long-term planning. For people with ADHD, saving up can be difficult because of their expectation of big results immediately. Even if they had a savings account, they would likely use up those savings quickly because they were short on groceries today.
- **Not taking shopping lists to the store** - Going shopping without a definitive list can be disastrous for those who like to spend as it can lead to impulse buying. Instead of quickly picking up a pint of milk and some bread, it ends up being a tub of ice cream, a few bags of chips, some sodas, and a few candies. A list helps set limits, so you don't overspend.
- **Taking out high-interest loans** - Risky financial behavior is an attribute of ADHD in adults. This could be in the form of taking out a loan without considering the long-term implications of doing so. This is attributed to a miscommunication in the pre-

frontal cortex, where impulsivity and decision-making are regulated.

The role impulsivity plays in overspending

Impulsivity greatly impacts financial struggles in adults with ADHD. Impulsivity can be emotional, action, or cognition. Adults with ADHD can, for example, go on a shopping spree (impulsivity of action) because of their bad day and get something to cheer them up (emotional impulsivity). This is the classic 'do now and think later' thinking associated with cognitive impulsivity. This is in no way, shape, or form a reflection of how irresponsible you are. The pre-frontal cortex that controls impulses and blocks out inappropriate actions isn't as strong in people with ADHD. That said, this is not to say you can't do anything about it. You can certainly improve your relationship with money.

How ADHD makes money more complicated for women

The numbers don't lie. Recent research indicates that women with ADHD are significantly more affected in managing their finances compared to men. 72% of women believe that their ADHD affects their finances more than 56% of men. Additionally, 80% of women with ADHD experience anxiety due to money problems caused by the disorder. Research found that women with ADHD are more likely to go on impulse shopping sprees than men. About 54% of women with ADHD say they do this often, while only 40% of men do. And that's not all; they also struggle more with sticking to a budget. 59% of them say it's a constant problem, while only 39% of guys feel the same way.

So, I guess the real question is, why does ADHD seem to hit women's financial management harder than men's? Well, women with ADHD tend to report more difficulties in various aspects of life, including managing money. It could be because of societal expectations. Women might view their financial abilities as weaker due to stereotypes that say women and people with ADHD can't handle their lives as well as others. It's possible that these negative perceptions could impact the self-evaluation of their financial skills.

FINANCIAL MANAGEMENT

As a woman with ADHD, managing your finances is vital, and you can do this through financial planning. Wouldn't it be nice not to worry about money and feel organized financially? Think about how great it would be to not get your phone service cut off because you forgot to pay your bill, or not being turned down for a loan. It's all within your reach.

Your relationship with money

If you're an adult with ADHD, there are a few things that might make it harder to keep up with your finances, such as:

- Finding it tough to keep track of your bank balances and expenses
- Organizing bills, checks, and tax papers

- Avoiding late payments
- Overspending and ending up with huge credit card balances
- Avoiding bill payments or putting off organizing financial records
- Difficulty saving up for an emergency fund or large purchase

Know where your money is going

If you're having trouble with impulsive spending, keeping a record of what you buy can really help. It'll also help you see where your money is going. All you need to do is grab a notebook or find a smartphone app that works for you and record all your purchases, even the small ones. Don't forget to include online purchases too.

When you track your spending, you'll start to notice certain categories popping up. These could include things like groceries, eating out, coffee shops, books, movies, gas, clothes, donations, and hobbies. It might first seem like a pain but stick with it for a week or two. If you're married or have a partner, they should do it too, so you can compare notes. If you're single, ask a trusted friend or family member to check in to ensure you're keeping track.

Even if you don't keep a perfect record of every expense, the information you do collect will help you improve your money management habits. Remember to include both fixed and variable expenses in your tracking. Fixed expenses generally cost the same amount each month. Examples of fixed expenses include rent, loans, or a car payment. Variable expenses are those expenses that can change every month. Examples of variable expenses include food, gas, clothing, and entertainment.

Make sure you include monthly, quarterly, and yearly expenses like taxes, homeowner association fees, and memberships. Once you add up your fixed and variable expenses, if they total more than your income, you'll need to look for ways to save or cut things out. Whatever's left over is your disposable income. You can use this for things like going out to dinner, making home repairs, taking vacations, or saving for retirement. It's up to you!

Think about your values and goals

Take a second and think about what you want to do short-term and long-term. If you're in a relationship, it's also a good idea to chat with your partner about your plans. It might help jot down some notes or create a picture board of things you want to save up for. Split your list or images into two groups - things you really need, like health, safety, or happiness, and things you want but don't necessarily need. Think about which things are the most important to you in both categories and what's stopping you from getting to where you want to be.

Once you figure out what you want and what's standing in your way, you can start making money goals. Short-term goals could be saving some cash each week or cutting back on eating out. Mid-term goals could be saving for a nice vacation or paying off a small debt. Long-term goals could be saving for college or preparing for retirement.

Break your goals down into small steps that you can work on daily, weekly, monthly, or yearly. And don't be afraid to ask for help if you need it. A friend, therapist, or coach can give you a hand. Just remember that being good with your money means always keeping your goals in mind. They're essential to your money management.

Curb impulse spending

We've all been there - you see something that catches your eye online, and in you go down the rabbit hole. Before you know it, you've spent much more than you planned, from small things like a pack of gum or a big-ticket item like a new laptop. Taking some time to learn how to control those impulses can really pay off for your budget and savings account. Here are a few tips to help you curb your impulse spending:

- **Figure out what your spending triggers are and try to avoid them**. Maybe a sale sign in a shop window or online is your Achilles' heel. Knowing your problem areas can help you stay away from temptation.
- **Make a shopping list and stick to it**. Before you head out to the store, write down everything you

need to buy, and don't let yourself get sidetracked. It might help to share your list with a friend or partner to keep yourself accountable.

- **Keep track of your spending as you go**. Adding up your purchases in real-time can help you stay aware of how much you're spending and avoid going over budget. You can consider putting a daily limit on your debit card to help you curb your spending. This way, you focus on getting the important stuff because of the spending limit.
- **Before making a big purchase, wait - maybe a day or two - to think it over**. If you still really want the item and have the money for it after that time has passed, then go ahead and buy it.
- **Unsubscribe from all those marketing emails that clutter up your inbox**. They're just trying to get you to spend money!
- **Look for fun, free, or low-cost hobbies and activities to keep yourself busy.** Check out local museums, parks, and libraries, or try joining a sports league or club.
- **Make it harder for yourself to spend money**. Try leaving your cards and checkbook at home, or only bring as much cash as you need for the day.

Manage credit cards and debt

Let's talk about credit card debt. It can be a slippery slope that leads to some pretty bad financial situations, especially if you're not paying off your bills. The interest, late fees, and over-the-limit charges can turn small purchases into big expenses that could take you up to 30 years to pay off! So, next time you're thinking about spending, ask yourself if you really want to be paying it off for the next 30 years. Credit cards are easy to use, but they also make it easy to spend more money than you have. If you're struggling with credit card debt, it might be a good idea to freeze them in a container of water so that you must wait and really think about whether you want to make the purchase.

Some other ideas for cutting back on your credit card use include:

- Having a friend or family member hold onto your card so that you need to have a conversation before making any purchases
- Writing a check for the amount of the purchase as soon as you make it
- Putting a sticker on your card to remind you of your long-term goals and help you pause before making purchases that don't fit with those goals.

Getting rid of debt and preventing new debt is the key to financial success. If you're struggling with credit card debt, consider meeting with a financial advisor to come up with a plan. And don't be afraid to talk to your therapist about any emotional issues you have around money. You've got this!

SAVING AND SPENDING

Savings are like a good raincoat you can put on, on a rainy day. It's like having your own personal safety net for whatever life throws your way. Maybe it's an unexpected expense, or maybe it's a big, exciting purchase you've been dreaming of, but having savings gives you the peace of mind that you're covered. If you're just starting with saving, don't worry if it feels tough at first. You can start small and work your way up as you get the hang of it. One idea is to open up a savings account specifically for this purpose - you could even set up automatic deposits from your paycheck, so you don't even have to think about it. If you really want to challenge yourself, try not to even have a debit card for that account, just to make sure you're only using the money for what you intended.

To make saving even more fun, make it visual and exciting. Maybe make a colorful chart with a thermometer-style tracker to watch your savings grow or create a cool bar graph on your computer that you update regularly. And for short-term goals, try putting cash in a jar or envelope with a picture of what you're saving for on the outside; every time you add money, you'll be reminded of why you're doing it!

Develop a spending plan

Creating a spending plan, or budget can be a helpful tool in preparing for your monthly or yearly expenses. It allows you to plan for recurring bills like utilities and loan installments and helps you avoid impulsive spending. To get started, write down how much money you need each month and consider using a spreadsheet to help organize your spending plan. There are many ways to create a budget that works for you, but here are some suggestions to get you started:

- Make a master list of all your expected expenses by pulling together amounts from purchases you made during the last 12 months
- Use money management programs like Quicken or Mint to help organize your spending information or consider using an Excel spreadsheet
- Add up all the expenses from the past 12 months and divide them by 12 to get your total average monthly expenses
- Set aside a regular day each week to review your spending plan and budget and determine which bills or expenses you expect for the coming week
- Consider paying bills online or setting up automatic payments to make the process easier
- Open a savings account and make regular deposits to cover sudden emergencies and save for special items or events
- Create a financial calendar or timeline to keep track of your bills and expenses

Creating a budget is a process and it may take some time to find what works best for you. Be patient with yourself and celebrate your progress as you develop this important financial habit.

Create a timeline

Some people like to break down their money management into a timeline that shows what financial tasks they need to do and how often they should do them. By doing this, you can see how quickly and easily some tasks can be completed, which can motivate you to get them done.

You can create your own timeline based on your goals and lifestyle. Here's an example of a timeline:

Every day

- Collect receipts from your wallet, car, desk drawer, or other places *(5 minutes)*
- Enter receipts and expenditures in your personal finance software (Quicken, Mint, You Need a Budget, etc.
- Keep receipts in an envelope until the end of the month *(5 minutes)*
- Open bills that came in the mail, and write the date each one needs to be mailed
- Keep all your bills somewhere you'll see them often *(5 minutes)*

Once a week

- Pay bills and keep records of them *(10 minutes)*
- Look through your email or apps for notifications of automatic bill payments made from your account that week and enter them in your personal finance software or checkbook *(10 minutes)*
- Review your expenses for the week that just ended and any you expect in the coming week *(5 minutes)*
- Deposit checks and withdraw money for the week *(time depends on the distance to your bank)*
- Consider creating an envelope for impulse spending so you have a set amount you allow yourself to spend *(5 minutes)*
- Review your weekly spending, especially in areas where you have a history of saving or spending difficulties *(10-15 minutes)*

Once a month

- Balance your bank statement *(20 minutes)*
- Discard or shred ATM receipts, debit receipts, and other receipts from the period covered by the most recent bank statement *(10 minutes)*
- Look over your budget and compare your goals to your actual spending and saving *(15 minutes)*
- Look for patterns in your spending habits so you can work to change them *(15 minutes)*

Once a year

- Collect your financial papers for tax filing, including any tax forms you receive in the mail from your employer, bank, mortgage lender, investment firms, college or university, etc., as well as records of any charitable donations *(20 minutes)*
- File your taxes or bring your information to a tax preparer *(time depends on whether you complete your taxes yourself)*
- Look over your spending and saving for the past year and make an honest assessment of how you did in meeting your goals *(30-45 minutes)*
- List any large expenses you may be facing in the coming year so you can start saving for them *(30 minutes)*
- Make a list of your ongoing debts, including how much you still owe and when you expect to pay each one off *(30-45 minutes)*

AVOID IMPULSIVE SPENDING

We've talked about how impulsive spending can negatively impact your finances. Here are some simple tips to help you gain control over impulsive spending and keep your finances in better order.

Learn of your impulsive spending

The first step in changing this behavior is simply recognizing that there's a behavior that needs changing. For example, if you're struggling with uncontrolled spending, acknowledging that it's a problem is a big step in the right direction. Once you're aware of the issue, you'll be better equipped to make a plan and stick to it.

Make shopping lists

We've already discussed how shopping lists can help keep you from overspending. This cannot be overstated. It's easy to forget what you wanted to buy when there are so many options staring you in the face.

Use cash rather than credit cards

As we've seen, credit cards can be a convenient way to make purchases, but they can also be risky when it comes to impulsive spending. To avoid this, consider using cash instead. It's harder to part with your cash and easier to keep track of your spending.

Delay the impulse to spend

Shop on an empty wallet or bring your designated impulse spending envelope. Take the time to browse and window shop to find exactly what you need. Once you've found the item, ask the salesperson to hold it for a day. This gives you time to go home, reflect, and ask yourself if you really need the item and if you can afford it. This approach can help you avoid impulse purchases and ensure that you're making the right decision for your budget.

Keep tags on purchases

In case you do end up making a purchase, consider keeping the tags on the item for a day or two. If the item comes in a sealed box, try not to open it right away. This gives you some time to really think about the purchase and make sure it's the right decision. You can always return it if you decide it was an impulse buy. This approach can help you avoid buyer's remorse and ensure you're making purchases you're delighted with.

Shop online

If you're looking for something specific, it's best to avoid the mall and try shopping online instead. When you find a few options you like, add them to your cart, and then take a few days to think about your decision. This gives you time to reflect and decide whether the items are really what you need and want. By taking this approach, you can avoid being tempted by other items at the mall and ensure you're making a thoughtful purchase that you'll be happy with in the long run.

Discuss major purchases before buying

Before making a major purchase and spending a ton of money, consider discussing it with someone you trust - your spouse, a friend, or a family member. They can help you weigh the pros and cons and decide whether it's a wise decision to make. Talking it through with someone can also provide you with a fresh perspective and help you avoid making impulsive decisions.

Don't shop socially

The mall is a popular spot to hang out with friends and have a good time while shopping. However, it's important to be mindful of the shopping frenzy that can happen when we're surrounded by our friends. It's easy to get caught up in the excitement and make purchases we don't really need, especially when our friends are telling us how great something looks. To avoid overspending in this situation, try to stay focused on your needs and budget. And if you do end up making a purchase, make sure it's something you truly want and need, and not just because your friends think it looks cool.

Learn to say no

The key to avoiding overspending is to focus on your needs, rather than wants. It's easy to get caught up in the excitement of shopping and fall into the trap of thinking, "I must have this." In the long run, this behavior can have negative repercussions, like debt and financial stress. So, take a step back and ask yourself if you really need the item, or if it's just a want. By being mindful of your spending and focusing on your true needs, you can avoid the negative consequences of overspending.

SUMMARY

- Adults with ADHD may struggle to manage their finances because of attention and impulse control difficulties
- People with ADHD have a higher propensity for getting into debt, spending impulsively, and taking out high-interest loans
- The pre-frontal cortex that controls impulses and blocks out inappropriate actions isn't as strong in people with ADHD, which greatly impacts impulsivity in spending
- ADHD impacts women's financial management harder than men's because of societal expectations
- Evaluate your relationship with money and know where your money goes
- Create a budget and avoid things that cause you to spend impulsively.
- Save as much as you can and spend less

ADHD can affect your relationship with money, leading to impulsive spending and poor financial management. This can also spill over into your living space, resulting in clutter and messiness. Therefore, it's important to develop strategies to not only manage finances but living environment too. Let's turn our attention to having a more livable home.

6

A MORE LIVABLE HOME

CLITTER-CLUTTER

I love my home, but my friends always joke that it's always just full of stuff. I mean, I collect trinkets, and I enjoy displaying them around the place. But I've been told it's actually cluttered. Interesting observation, given that I recently read about hoarding and OCD. I'm trying to take on board what I read. The paper talked about Hoarding Disorder (HD) being a condition that is often not recognized or treated properly. It usually develops during early adulthood, but people tend to seek help only later in life. Unfortunately, this means that research on HD is mostly based on older women. While HD was previously thought to be related to Obsessive-Compulsive Disorder (OCD), it is now understood that individuals with HD may also experience symptoms similar to those of ADHD.

It's interesting to know that historically, there has been a connection between HD and OCD, as seen in the way they're classified and researched. It's also worth noting that recent studies and clinical observations suggest a possible link between HD and ADHD. Individuals with ADHD can struggle with attention and impulsivity, and this can persist into adulthood, causing functional difficulties. Similarly, people with HD also face challenges with attention, processing information, and executive functioning. In fact, individuals with OCD have shown that those with HD are more likely to have ADHD, particularly the inattentive subtype.

ADHD AND MESSINESS

If you have ADHD, you might have experienced how the disorder affects your mind and physical surroundings. It's like a chaotic tornado that wreaks havoc on your space, making it impossible to keep things neat and tidy. You may have wondered if messiness is just a quirk of your personality or a direct result of your ADHD, and most importantly if anything can be done to help you get organized.

A prevalence of messiness has been found in people with ADHD, why it happens, and some strategies that can help you tidy up your space. Let's get to it.

Can ADHD cause you to be messy and disorganized?

Working memory is a type of short-term memory that helps us remember recent information for tasks we're currently working on. If you struggle with working memory, it can impact your organizational skills and make it tough to plan and follow through on tasks towards a goal. This could mean having trouble organizing your physical space, like your home or office. For instance, you might have clean laundry sitting unfolded on the floor for days or start multiple creative projects but leave them unfinished and cluttering up your space. Misplacing items could also be a common occurrence.

It's worth noting that disorganization isn't a universal symptom for those with ADHD, and some people find that treatment and management strategies can help them get more organized. It's also possible to struggle with being disorganized without having ADHD due to other factors like a busy schedule or a lack of interest in tidiness. It's important to keep in mind that additional symptoms beyond being forgetful or disorganized are needed to get an ADHD diagnosis.

DECLUTTERING

If you're an adult with ADHD and you've got a messy workspace or a chaotic home, don't worry too much. If you're finding yourself buried under piles of stuff, it's time to take action and learn how to keep the clutter from taking over your life.

There is a debate among ADHD experts regarding whether a cluttered environment suggests a genius mind. I tend to align with the belief that clutter is a sign of brilliance. Still, the truth may vary from person to person and the extent of their organizational challenges. Individuals who struggle with organization may devote excessive time to tidying their surroundings, compromising on quality time with family and friends. For ADHD adults, a state of controlled chaos may be a more feasible alternative. Nevertheless, if the clutter is left unchecked, it can escalate and become overwhelming.

Messy and organized

The most important factor to consider when dealing with clutter is not the opinions of others, but rather how you personally feel about it and how it impacts your productivity. As an adult with ADHD, you may find that you can perform just as well in a cluttered environment at home or work, despite being labeled a slob by others. Some of the most disorganized people have an uncanny ability to locate a specific document from a towering stack of papers without any difficulty. To me, that's a sign of true organization, regardless of the mess. It's more fulfilling to live up to your own expectations than to force yourself to conform to the standards of those with an innate talent for sorting.

Relatives, friends, and colleagues may criticize you for your clutter and view you as lazy or disorganized, even if this isn't true. If you feel in control of your mess and it's not impeding your ability to function, don't let the criticism get to you. To determine whether you're in control, ask yourself questions like, "Am I wasting time searching for things I need?" or "Am I being sidetracked by clutter, resulting in minimal progress?" If you answer these questions negatively, you may have a mess you can live with.

Messy and dysfunctional

ADHD adults may be able to recognize the signs that their clutter is taking over their lives. There are seven unmistakable indicators:

- Replacing lost items that have been buried in clutter
- Spending valuable time searching for frequently used objects
- Receiving complaints from a spouse or co-worker about the clutter infringing on their personal space
- Being distracted by the mess on one's desk
- Being told by a supervisor to tidy up one's workspace
- Finding items in incorrect locations, such as dishes in the bedroom or clothes in the dining room
- Having a pile of papers that topples over or having to step over things to navigate through a room

Don't let clutter overwhelm you

When managing clutter and staying organized; it's important to remember that perfection is not the goal. While having a clean and organized space can certainly be helpful, it's not the only measure of success. If you're overwhelmed by clutter, becoming critical of yourself, and your abilities can be easy. However, it's important to take a step back and recognize that you have many positive qualities that are unrelated to your ability to stay organized.

Rather than focusing solely on your clutter, find something about yourself to applaud. Perhaps you're a great listener, a skilled problem solver, or a creative thinker. Maybe you're a loyal friend, a dedicated employee, or a loving partner. By focusing on your strengths and positive qualities, you can build your self-esteem and feel more confident in yourself. This, in turn, can help you tackle clutter and stay organized with a more positive and optimistic mindset.

It's also important to remember that clutter and disorganization are not personal failings. Many people struggle with clutter and disorganization, and it does not reflect on your worth as a person. You can progress towards being more organized by taking small steps to tackle your clutter and seeking support when needed.

ADHD-FRIENDLY WAYS OF GETTING ORGANIZED

Life is unpredictable, and what works today might not work tomorrow. But the good news is that even small changes and some ADHD organization tools can make a big difference. You'll have less clutter, fewer headaches, and more peace of mind. So, it's worth giving it a shot!

1. Set time limits for decision-making

Individuals with ADHD can sometimes take longer to make decisions that others make in a snap. It can be super frustrating, but there are ways to speed up the process. One trick is to set a time limit or a budget limit. Let's say you're trying to find the perfect summer camp for your kid. Give yourself a deadline to make the decision and do the best you can with the options you have by that date. Or, if you're trying to pick a new phone, set a maximum price you're willing to pay and ignore the fancier, pricier options.

Another tip is to figure out the most important factor for making the decision. Is it the price, convenience, style, practicality, or something else? Once you've figured that out, focus solely on that factor when making your choice. It'll make the decision-making process a whole lot easier and less overwhelming.

2. Fight the tendency to overcommit

If you have ADHD, it's easy to get overwhelmed with too many commitments. One helpful tip is to make a trade-off: for every new thing you agree to do, give up something else. For example, let's say you decide to join the school fundraising committee. To avoid spreading yourself too thin, consider giving up another commitment, like being part of the neighborhood watch committee. Doing this lets you focus on the new commitment without adding more to your plate.

Remember, adults with ADHD tend to take on too much, so it's important to be mindful of your limits and not over-commit yourself. By making smart trade-offs like this, you can stay more organized and avoid feeling overwhelmed.

3. Keep your to-do lists brief

MAKE A TO-DO LIST!

- Use BIG, BOLD letters
- Only list FIVE tasks on an index card
- If you have more tasks, put them on the back of the card
- Once you finish those five things, use the back of the card to make a NEW list
- Throw away the old list

By following these simple steps, you'll get more done, feel less frustrated, and manage your time like a boss. So, go ahead, grab an index card, and get to work.

4. Fight hyperfocus

If you're the kind of person who easily gets sucked down the rabbit hole and gets lost with social media for hours on end, it's time to get some help. Set your phone alarm or kitchen timer to remind you when it's time to stop scrolling and move on to something else. Or, if you prefer, you could arrange for a reliable friend or family member to give you a call at a certain time to snap you out of it.

5. Keep extra medication on hand

Every time you fill a prescription, make sure to mark it in your planner when you need to renew it. You could also set up an alert on your computer or have an email reminder generated on that date. To make things even easier, ask your pharmacist if they can give you a call or text to remind you when it's time to refill. Make sure to set your "renew date" at least one week before you run out of your medication to avoid any lapses. By staying on top of your medication schedule, you'll be able to stay healthy and focused on the important things in life.

6. Build socializing into your schedule

If you're looking to meet new people, enjoy some interesting conversations, and keep up with friends without any hassle, you can get involved in a class, outdoor club, book club, lecture series, or start your own dinner club! By participating in these activities, you'll be able to expand your social circle, learn new things, and have fun without worrying about making plans or scheduling meetups. Go ahead and sign up for that class you've been eyeing or start a club with your closest friends. Trust me, it's an easy and enjoyable way to stay socially active!

7. Join an ADHD support group

Did you know that support groups can provide more than just emotional support? For example, members can come together online to tackle boring tasks like filling out tax returns or filing. One person takes a turn and dedicates 15 minutes to the task at hand while others continue to chat through instant messaging. Once the task is completed, the person returns to the group, and they all congratulate each other, joke around, and share their experiences.

8. Stop agonizing over insignificant items

If you've got a bunch of greeting cards, batteries with questionable power, unidentified cords, and other random items that you're not sure what to do with, designate a "ripening drawer" to toss them into. When the drawer is full, take some time to quickly sort through everything. Keep what you can use and discard the rest. Then, start the process again by filling the drawer with new items. This simple trick can help you avoid cluttering up your living space with items you don't need or use.

9. Get a clutter companion

Get a nonjudgmental friend or family member to help you declutter your home. Sort items into four piles: "keep," "toss," "donate," and "age." Get rid of the "toss" items right away. Put "donate" items in sturdy garbage bags and take them to the nearest donation center. Put "age" items in a labeled cardboard box with a date three months ahead. Mark the same date in your calendar as a reminder to review the items in the box. If you're ready to discard them, do so; otherwise, set a new date to review them again in three months.

10. Get rid of pile-ups

To effectively manage magazine clutter, it's best to limit yourself to a small basket no larger than six inches in height and two magazine widths across to store unread issues. Once the basket is full, go through the magazines and read what you can. Discard or recycle the rest or donate them to a hospital or women's shelter.

For loose change, keep a jar within reach and drop in coins that accumulate on your dresser. At the end of the month, you can use the money you've saved as a reward for keeping your pockets clutter-free.

If you tend to keep mail and bills for months, look at what you really need for tax purposes or to keep for your records. Put those papers in a folder and toss out the rest.

11. Make use of "wasted" minutes

Rather than waiting for lengthy periods of uninterrupted time to tackle organizational tasks, it's helpful to use even short amounts of time productively. For instance, in just one minute, you could accomplish small tasks like sorting through your mail, removing lint from the dryer, or watering your plants. If you have five minutes available, you could empty the dishwasher or draft a quick email. Even when waiting for laundry to finish, you could use that time to match up socks or gather clothes for dry cleaning.

12. Organize your wardrobe

When you have a large wardrobe, it can be challenging to decide what to wear each morning. To simplify the process, it's useful to regularly remove any excess clothing. If you purchase a new shirt, for example, consider donating or selling an older one. During the spring and summer, focus on coordinating your outfits around two main colors plus white. Similarly, during the fall and winter, coordinate your clothing around two other colors and black. This approach allows you to have a more manageable number of outfits to choose from, which saves you both time and money.

Try using sturdy hangers to hang your clothes in the closet will help you get dressed more quickly and with less confusion. This approach works well for both men and women, particularly for organizing business attire. Women may find attaching a baggie containing matching jewelry to the hanger helpful. Consider using a days-of-the-week closet organizer for organizing children's clothes and toys.

13. Pick the right time of day

Not all of us are morning people, especially those with ADHD. However, there's no rule stating that you must work in the morning. If you're more productive at night, don't hesitate to try! Experiment with different times of the day to see what works best for you.

14. Take before, and after pictures

People with ADHD often struggle with accurately assessing their progress and time management skills. Taking "before" and "after" photos of your progress is important. You don't need to share them with anyone. These photos can serve as a visual reminder of your achievements and motivate you to keep going. You'll realize just how far you've come when you compare them. Celebrate your accomplishments with your favorite beverage or a relaxing evening. You deserve it!

SUMMARY

- ADHD can affect your working memory, which can impact your organizational skills
- Some people spend too much time organizing their environment, which can lead to less time with loved ones
- Adults with ADHD may find it more practical to embrace a state of controlled chaos
- As an adult with ADHD, you may find that you can perform just as well in a cluttered environment
- You can get yourself organized by being deliberate and strategic

You may struggle with organization and may find it easier to work in a state of controlled chaos. But this can be challenging in a work environment that values structure and order. Therefore, it's important to develop strategies to manage symptoms and succeed at work. Let's look at ADHD at work.

7

ADHD AT WORK

UPSIDE-DOWN ETHIC

So interesting fact - more than half of surveyed adults with ADHD said they lost or changed jobs because of their ADHD symptoms. Crazy, right? And get this - over 36% had 4 or more jobs in the past 10 years, and 6.5% had 10 or more jobs in the same period. The ADHD Awareness Coalition says finding the right job and asking for minor accommodations can help succeed in the workplace. I'm floored. It's crazy that people like me with ADHD haven't held down jobs. I think it's this ableist society with its lack of accommodation. Why should we have to ask for accommodation? I would think it's something that should be ingrained in company culture. All this talk of diversity is cheap if people with ADHD are the ones making the most accommodations to try to fit in the world of work.

It's pretty nuts because millions of people live with ADHD in America alone. That's a good chunk of the population. Perhaps employers need to reevaluate their policies on people with ADHD in the workplace. I think if an employee has ADHD, the HR department can get an expert to help them out and make sure they get the support they need. I'm curious to see how this unfolds over time.

SYMPTOMS POSING PROBLEMS IN THE WORKPLACE

As an adult with ADHD, work can become a real challenge. It's not uncommon to experience difficulties completing tasks, arriving at work on time, or meeting deadlines. This can often lead to missing out on promotions, being let go from jobs, or struggling to get along with colleagues.

Which adult ADHD symptoms pose problems in the workplace?

ADHD symptoms can cause difficulties at work, regardless of the type of job or workplace. Some of the most challenging symptoms include the following:

- Getting easily bored with tasks or projects
- Struggling with distractions caused by both internal and external stimuli
- Forgetting tasks or deadlines
- Being unable to sit still due to hyperactivity

- Making impulsive decisions without considering consequences
- Having poor relationship skills, such as interrupting others or being too blunt
- Struggling with time management, including meeting deadlines and estimating task completion time
- Procrastinating by putting off tasks

SHOULD YOU LET THEM KNOW?

Your friends and family may know about your ADHD, but your colleagues and superiors at work don't. So, the question is, should you disclose your condition to your boss? It's a tricky decision, and the right solution varies depending on your work circumstances. Will your disclosure be met with understanding and support, or it could make things tougher for you at work? It's important to know that you do not have to share information about your ADHD with anyone at work. Here are a few considerations to help you make this decision:

Your legal rights

Americans with Disabilities Act (ADA) is there to protect people with disabilities from workplace discrimination, and this applies to all types of jobs, including government and private employers with 15 employees or more. ADA also protects people with ADHD, but you've got to show, with proper documentation, that your ADHD is affecting your work. If you meet the requirements, your boss has to work with you to find ways to help you do your job better.

Pros and cons

If you open up to your boss about your ADHD, they may be more likely to work with you to find accommodations that help you thrive. Sharing the challenges of your ADHD can help your employer and colleagues better understand your needs, your work style, and how to collaborate with you more effectively. In a perfect world, employers recognize the advantages of working with employees who have ADHD, but of course, we don't live in a perfect world. Your boss may not understand ADHD and may be hesitant to make any extra effort to accommodate you.

Things to consider

When deciding whether to tell your boss about your ADHD, it's important to consider your goals. What do you hope to achieve by having this conversation? It's also worth considering whether there are other ways to meet your needs without disclosing your ADHD. Every situation is unique, so it's important to simulate and plan for possible outcomes. Consider your relationship with your boss as well. Is it positive and supportive, or is there tension between you? Also, think about your performance at work. If you're generally a strong performer struggling due to ADHD, you may be more likely to receive help and understanding. Unfortunately, those already struggling with poor performance and relationships may have a harder time getting the support they need.

Consider your company and the industry you're in

Some companies are great about embracing diversity and differences among their employees, while others may expect everyone to fit a certain mold. It can be tough to know where your company falls on that spectrum. To help you decide, there are a few questions you can ask yourself. Have other employees with ADHD disclosed their condition and had a positive experience? Does your company offer mental health programs and accommodations for employees with disabilities or challenges? How much does your company know about ADHD, and is their information accurate?

Also consider your industry and your own expertise. If your skills are in high demand, you may feel more comfortable disclosing your condition, as you could quickly find another job if needed. But if your industry is small or highly competitive, disclosing might impact your job opportunities in the future.

The middle ground

If you're considering talking to your boss about your work challenges, experts suggest focusing on those specific challenges rather than bringing up ADHD right away. This approach isn't meant to be deceptive but to help your employer better understand your obstacles and how to address them for a positive outcome. The same goes for your co-workers - explaining how certain distractions or interruptions affect your work and what you need to be successful is helpful.

Think of it like a sales pitch: you're presenting an opportunity to increase productivity and ultimately benefit the company's bottom line. To make the conversation productive, you can use a three-step approach: first, highlight the struggle and circumstances; second, bring a solution; and third, describe the benefits of that solution for the company.

Choosing not to share

If you feel that the risks of disclosing your ADHD outweigh the benefits, it's okay to keep it to yourself. Take the necessary steps to clearly understand how ADHD specifically affects your job performance. This way, you can work through the issues with help from an ADHD coach or training program that focuses on addressing workplace challenges. There are resources out there to support you in achieving success at work; make use of them!

Note that asking for accommodations does not necessarily mean you'll get them. Some employers believe that providing accommodations for their employees could be costly or create an appearance of bias towards certain individuals. Some may approve accommodations for their employees but fail to make them accessible or feasible.

MANAGING SYMPTOMS AT WORK

A survey found that adults with ADHD can face challenges keeping full-time jobs and earn less than their peers without the disorder. ADHD can affect job performance in various ways, such as difficulty with attention, working memory, and executive-function abilities that are important in the workplace. People with ADHD may also have trouble with time management (which we'll discuss later), staying organized, completing assignments, and controlling their emotions, which can lead to feelings of depression and low self-esteem.

How can you get and keep a job

If you're starting a job search, consider working with a career counselor or a coach to help you find a job that suits your interests, needs, and abilities. Maybe you'll prefer a more fast-paced job with flexible hours or even starting your own business to create your ideal work environment. The possibilities are endless!

Here are ways you can stay organized and focused once you have landed your job:

- **Find a quiet space** to work where distractions will be minimized. You could consider asking to be placed in a quiet area or requesting noise-canceling headphones to help you focus.

- **Buddy up.** Collaborate with a colleague or manager who possesses excellent organizational skills and can guide you throughout the project.
- **Book it** by keeping a planner to manage your schedule, tasks, appointments, and deadlines. Use electronic reminders on your phone or computer to help you stay on top of your commitments.
- **Write it down.** During meetings and phone calls, make sure to take notes and include any new tasks on your to-do list.
- **Schedule interruptions.** Allocate dedicated time to review your emails and voicemails, ensuring they do not disrupt your other tasks.
- **Set realistic goals.** Break your day into individual assignments and tackle one task at a time.
- **Reward yourself.** After completing a task, reward yourself with a break or a small treat.
- **Delegate.** Consider getting an assistant or intern to help with small details so you can focus on the big picture.
- **Relax.** Practice relaxation techniques such as deep breathing or meditation. Take breaks throughout the day to walk or talk to a coworker.
- **Seek guidance.** Talk to your career counselor or executive coach to help you navigate any issues or difficult situations you encounter on the job.

The Positive Side Of ADHD At Work

Since ADHD is classified as a disability by the Americans with Disabilities Act, it is prohibited for larger companies to discriminate against individuals based on their condition. The Act also mandates employers to make reasonable accommodations for employees with ADHD. This, therefore, means disclosing your ADHD diagnosis to your employer is crucial for them to provide the necessary support. Make sure you are well-prepared before talking to them.

Attributes of ADHD, such as restlessness, impulsivity, and a constant desire for novelty, make it an asset in certain contexts, such as entrepreneurship. Many studies have shown that individuals with ADHD are more likely to become successful entrepreneurs. The key is to identify a career that aligns with your strengths and use your energy, creativity, and other attributes to excel in your job.

TIME WASTERS AND PRODUCTIVITY KILLERS

Time wasters and productivity killers are activities or behaviors that consume time without adding value to one's work or personal life. They can range from small distractions like checking social media, chatting with colleagues, or browsing the internet to more significant distractions like attending unnecessary meetings, procrastinating on important tasks, or engaging in low-priority work. Time wasters can be particularly challenging for individuals with ADHD, as they may struggle to prioritize tasks and resist distractions.

ADHD at Work

Are you struggling to be punctual at work? Do you experience challenges in staying focused and meeting deadlines, or find yourself fixating on minor details for extended periods? Maybe your desk is in disarray, and locating your phone proves difficult. While everyone faces job-related challenges, adults with ADHD face a constant battle with details that can result in conflict with managers, missed promotions, and a stagnant career. Studies reveal that college graduates with ADHD earn an average of $4,300 less per year than their neurotypical peers.

To excel at work despite having ADHD, it's important to customize your work environment. You can capitalize on your strengths, such as creativity or interpersonal skills, while mitigating the negative effects of your weaknesses.

ADHD and executive dysfunction

As we've discussed, poor executive functioning is a common challenge for individuals with ADHD. It can lead to various difficulties in the workplace, such as spending excessive time on a minor task or getting sidetracked by small interruptions, which can lead colleagues to perceive those with ADHD as disorganized, disruptive, or unproductive. Despite these challenges, people with ADHD often work harder than their colleagues to keep up with their workload. They may experience moments of brilliance interspersed with periods of difficulty focusing, which can be frustrating for both the individual and their colleagues. The fluctuations in attention and focus that individuals with ADHD experience may result in papers not getting filed and the office being messy, which, in this case, is not a sign of laziness or disorganization.

A two-pronged approach to ADHD at work

Individuals with ADHD often benefit from a combination of medication and counseling to develop effective strategies for addressing job-related challenges. Meeting the diagnostic criteria for ADHD, including hyperactivity, distractibility, or compulsive behavior in multiple settings, typically warrants the use of medication. With the right medication, individuals may experience an improved ability to focus on tasks, control impulsive behavior, and work productively.

Finding the appropriate ADHD medication is not enough. Ensuring the medication dosage schedule covers the full workday is crucial. For example, if an individual works from 7:30 am to 6:30 pm, taking an eight-hour pill before work may wear off around 3:30 pm, requiring the use of a four-hour pill at that time. If working from home, it may also be necessary to have coverage in the evening.

Ending ADHD distractions at work

To work at peak efficiency, it's crucial to develop a workplace strategy that minimizes distractions. One of the best ways to achieve this is to schedule work during quiet times, which can be achieved by arriving early to work. If possible, having a flexible schedule or a private office can also be helpful. But if this is not an option, it may be possible to work in an empty office or conference room to avoid interruptions. To minimize external distractions, it's important not to answer the phone, but let voicemail take messages and return calls later. A "Do Not Disturb" sign can also help deter interruptions. Facing the desk towards a wall and keeping the workplace free of clutter can help reduce visual distractions.

Be aware of internal distractions, such as lightbulb moments, sudden realizations of forgotten tasks, and daydreaming. To address these, jotting down creative ideas for later review, using a planning system, and finding more interesting work can be helpful. Solutions can also be tailored to specific problems, such as using a double-checklist system to ensure important steps are not missed. Setting cues such as Post-it notes, watch alarms, or pop-up boxes can be helpful for those prone to hyperfocus. For individuals with hyperactivity, taking breaks every hour for physical activity, such as light exercise that you can do in the office or a stroll through the halls, can also be beneficial.

Staying on schedule

To enhance productivity, individuals with ADHD may benefit from collaborating with a coworker or supervisor, as we mentioned earlier, to develop and monitor a detailed work schedule. To prevent disruptions to your schedule, avoid making impulsive commitments. Instead of automatically agreeing to requests, use a catchphrase such as "I'd like to, but let me check my calendar."

When commuting or going to an appointment, allocate extra time for travel. Rather than focusing on the arrival time, prioritize the time you need to leave your current location to arrive on schedule. Avoid the "just-one-more-thing" temptation. If you think of another task as you are about to leave, it's best to write it down and tackle it later.

TIME MANAGEMENT

As you are now aware, individuals with ADHD often experience significant difficulties with time management, which can lead to frustration and obstacles in completing tasks. Executive functions help us complete tasks we know we should do. But because individuals with ADHD tend to struggle with focusing on the future, they may find it difficult to engage in activities that will benefit them in the end. For instance, completing tomorrow's office assignment or implementing healthy habits now could prevent problems and illnesses later. Therefore, understanding and managing ADHD as a condition that affects time management can help.

ADHD is too much present, not enough future

Life can be overwhelming, with countless distractions vying for our attention and goals requiring our efforts. Some tasks are enjoyable, while others are tedious or frustrating. It's easy to get caught up in immediate rewards like a funny tweet, but balancing living in the moment with planning for the future is essential. However, it's challenging to disconnect from the present and create space to make the best decisions.

Individuals with ADHD find it particularly hard to prioritize future goals over the distractions of the present. As we've seen, they are easily absorbed by what's happening around them, making it challenging to plan for the future. Unlike neurotypicals, who can apply executive functions to make decisions based on their goals, people with ADHD struggle to prioritize long-term rewards or consequences. Deadlines or alarms set for the future don't always motivate them to act in the present.

Many adults with ADHD find it challenging to consider future events or consequences until it's too late. Even if a task is on their radar, they might not feel motivated to act on it. As a result, they rely heavily on deadlines to take action and often find themselves procrastinating until the last minute.

See time by externalizing it

Having ADHD may mean finding it difficult to understand time management and what needs to be done when. But that's totally fine! There are plenty of external tools that can help supplement internal abilities. For instance, having multiple analog clocks within easy view can make the passage of time more visible. It's important to be aware of what time it is and to intentionally make choices based on that knowledge.

To stay on track, stick to your scheduling system to help you get things done. If you have a lot of items on your schedule, setting reminders and alarms can help you stay on track. And if you put to-do list items into your schedule, you're more likely to actually complete them.

Scheduling tasks can also help you reduce over-commitment by letting you see your day filling up. Rather than having a long list of tasks to complete, block out chunks of time for each task. If something isn't completed or circumstances change, no worries! Just move it to a different time on your schedule. By seeing the big picture of your day, you can make better decisions about what needs to be done and when.

Feel time by maximizing motivation

For people with ADHD, it can be hard to feel the effects of their actions until it's too late, even if they know what they should be doing. It's tough to resist the present temptations when the future consequences don't feel real enough. For example, it's easy to say, "Let's eat out tonight, we'll save for retirement later." To make future consequences feel more real, you need to tap into your past experiences and bring that feeling to the present. Imagine how you'll feel in the future if you don't start working on something now. Try to envision it in as much detail as possible. Ask yourself questions like, "How will I feel on Thursday night if I start preparing for the Friday meeting now? How will I feel during the meeting? What if I wait until the last minute?" The more you can visualize the future and its consequences, the more motivated you'll be to take action.

Tip the balance

Managing your time effectively can be a slippery slope and unfamiliar, but it ultimately comes down to a battle between prioritizing the present and the future. The present will always seem more alluring, but it's important to make a conscious effort to keep your future goals in mind. When dealing with ADHD, it's crucial to prioritize the future over the present in order to effectively manage your time.

Practical ways for ADHD brains to see time

Here are some practical ways to help you manage your time more effectively:

- Post notes with the time you need to leave each room (bathroom, bedroom, kitchen) and make sure there's a clock in each room
- When scheduling appointments, factor in travel time and set an alarm to remind you to leave
- Take a few minutes at the beginning of the day to prioritize your tasks and plan when you'll work on them

- Use a timer to remind you to go to bed
- Limit your time online by using Internet-limiting devices like Circle
- Turn off auto-play on streaming services to see the current time between videos

Practical ways to be mindful of time

Let's now look at some practical ways to help you be mindful of time:

- Check in with your boss or coworkers often to avoid procrastination
- Tell someone else what you plan to do and ask them to check up on you and hold you accountable
- Break up big projects into smaller deadlines, for example, finish report by Sunday, and first draft by Wednesday
- Prioritize sleep, diet, and exercise to boost energy and productivity
- Reward yourself for completing tasks, for example, going out after doing the dishes
- Set a bedtime to motivate yourself to finish tasks earlier in the evening
- If procrastinating is costing you money, think about what you could do with the money you'll save by taking action sooner
- Have a routine. Having a routine can improve memory retention, especially if you establish both a

morning and nighttime routine
- When planning a task, try to estimate the amount of time it will take to complete it
- To ensure that you have more accurate timeframe, consider doubling or even tripling your original estimate to allow for unexpected obstacles or delays

SUMMARY

- ADHD symptoms can affect productivity at work and so employees with ADHD face challenges at work, such as missed deadlines and time management issues
- Disclosing your ADHD to your employer is not mandatory and should be done after careful consideration and preparation
- Find ways to help you keep up at work, such as working in a quiet space and scheduling
- Time wasters make it difficult to prioritize tasks and eliminate distractions
- Understanding and managing ADHD as a condition that affects time management can be useful when m

ADHD can affect individuals in the workplace, making it difficult to stay organized and focused. Yet building healthy relationships and social skills can help individuals with ADHD succeed in their careers, which is what we will discuss next.

8

CULTIVATING HEALTHY RELATIONSHIPS & DEVELOPING SOCIAL SKILLS

LOVE IS AN OPEN DOOR

I continue to be inspired by women like me, with ADHD, who are doing so well, especially when cultivating relationships. Women like Mel, who share their stories, are nothing short of brave and inspirational. Mel's story goes like this: As someone with ADHD, I tend to be passive and open, which can attract toxic people into my life without me even noticing. It's hard for me to push them away because I don't want to hurt their feelings. I love making friends with everyone and learning about their lives, but it can lead to attracting negative people. Recently, I've learned about setting boundaries and walking away when necessary. I met my best friend and husband, Justin, in an impulsive moment, and he's been my rock ever since. When he was diagnosed with cancer during nursing school, I focused all my energy on helping him fight it. We won, and things are mostly back to normal. We laugh every day, even when he puts the empty Brita back in the fridge.

Having ADHD doesn't close you off to love. It doesn't mean you can't have healthy and mutually beneficial relationships with friends or a partner. I am really encouraged by such stories and I know that my condition is not the end of the world. It's just something that's there, but it doesn't necessarily make my life less beautiful. On the contrary! It makes me beautiful and unique. I love me, and I have people around me who love me too!

MASTERING SOCIAL SKILLS

As you know, ADHD can sometimes make you act impulsively, be disorganized, sensitive, intense, emotional, or disruptive. This can make it hard to get along with parents, siblings, teachers, friends, coworkers, or partners. Basically, you sometimes struggle to regulate your actions and reactions, which makes relationships tense and fragile. That's why this section covers relationship issues specific to people with ADHD and those around them.

SOCIAL SKILLS IN ADULTS WITH ADHD

People with ADHD can struggle to socialize, making friends, and keeping relationships because of their inattention, impulsivity, and hyperactivity. This can really suck and even lead to mood and anxiety problems.

Overall impact of ADHD on social interactions

It's no surprise that people with ADHD often struggle in social situations. Having good social skills is super important for kids to grow and develop, but over 50% of kids with ADHD have trouble making friends. Unfortunately, adults with ADHD also struggle with socializing, which can lead to loneliness and a bunch of other problems.

To have a successful interaction with someone, you need to be attentive, responsible, and in control of your impulses. But people with ADHD often struggle with those things. Since ADHD is an "invisible disability," others might not understand why someone is behaving in a certain way and blame it on something else. This can lead to negative labels and social rejection, which can be really tough on a person's self-esteem. But with education and proper treatment, people with ADHD can learn strategies to improve their social skills and form positive relationships.

ADHD and the acquisition of social skills

When it comes to social skills, most people learn by watching others, copying behavior, practicing, and getting feedback. It's a process that usually starts during childhood and is sharpened through observation and peer feedback. However, children with ADHD often miss these crucial details and may struggle with social expectations as adults.

Social acceptance is like a spiral that can go up or down. Those with good social skills are usually rewarded with acceptance from others and encouraged to improve further. But for those with ADHD, the spiral tends to go down. Their lack of social skills leads to rejection, which then limits their chances to learn social skills, leading to even more rejection. This can include things like being avoided or rejected by others, which is quite hurtful.

What's tough is that people don't usually tell someone when they've made a social mistake. Pointing out someone's error is often seen as impolite. This means that people with ADHD are often left to figure out what they're doing wrong on their own. This can be tough, but with the right support and strategies, people with ADHD can improve their social skills and build more positive relationships.

Research on children with ADHD and social skills

Researchers have looked into the social challenges faced by children with ADHD and found that they struggle with making friends, maintaining relationships, and behaving appropriately in social situations. This problem doesn't go away as they get older either, and can really get in the way of their social lives as adults. At first, people thought that children with ADHD just didn't have the right social skills, so they tried training them in social skills groups. The therapist would teach the children specific social behaviors and then they would practice using them with each other. They would get feedback and encouragement to use these new skills in their daily lives.

But now, researchers think that the real issue might be that children with ADHD have trouble using the social skills they already have. This is because they struggle with the executive functions of the brain. So even if they know the right way to act, they might be unable to do it consistently. This is where medication can come in handy, as it helps improve those executive functions. While social skills training can help, it doesn't always translate to other settings like school or public places. But researchers have found that incorporating social skills training into a more intensive behavioral program, like a summer camp, can be helpful in making sure the gains made in social skills training stick.

Although there have been some studies that show social skills training can be effective, there hasn't been much research on whether it leads to better relationships and social lives for children with ADHD as they grow up. So, there's definitely more work to be done in this area.

Specific ADHD symptoms and social skills

Inattention

Here are some tips for identifying nuances and some challenges people with ADHD may face in social interactions:

- Check out your environment for clues to help decipher nuances

- Be observant of body language, tone of voice, behavior, or eye contact to interpret what someone is saying
- Look at someone's choice of words to better understand their underlying meaning
- Actions speak louder than words, so pay attention to what people do as well as what they say
- Find a guide to help you with this hidden language
- Learn to interpret polite behavior
- Be alert to what others are doing

Some challenges that people with ADHD may face in social interactions include:

- Missing important information due to a lapse in attention
- Experiencing difficulty understanding nuances and reading the room
- Difficulty paying attention to both the text of a conversation and the subtext
- Difficulty understanding what someone says may not be what they mean

Impulsivity

Being impulsive can cause problems in your relationships with others. People might think you don't care about them or their feelings because you say or do things without thinking about the consequences. It can also make it hard to have good conversations with others because you might interrupt them or just talk too much. If you have ADHD, being impulsive can be even harder to control. You might make bad decisions or act before you really think things through. This can lead to all kinds of problems, like spending too much money or getting into fights. Plus, if you talk really fast all the time, it can be hard for others to keep up with you and feel like they're a part of the conversation.

Hyperactivity

Individuals with ADHD often experience limitations in participating in leisure activities due to their physical hyperactivity. Their inability to sit still and concentrate during events such as concerts, religious ceremonies, educational activities, or vacations can appear to others as a lack of interest or concern. Moreover, their difficulty in appearing attentive can leave others feeling ignored or neglected.

Assessment of social skills

When a mental health professional wants to check if an adult has social skill deficits and interpersonal interaction problems related to ADHD, they usually use interviews and self-report questionnaires. It's part of the diagnostic evaluation process. The questionnaires are a means to collect information from a person with ADHD and from their friends or partners. They ask about things like how the person pays attention when spoken to, if they interrupt others a lot, or if they miss social cues. The questions cover different areas, like communication skills, manners, and staying organized. Some people with ADHD might also have trouble with noisy environments or get overwhelmed easily. They might have disorganized thoughts or talk a lot without staying on topic. Sometimes they might end conversations abruptly too.

How ADHD can positively affect social skills

Having ADHD comes with its own advantages. It can boost your social skills in several ways. People with ADHD can be really curious, enthusiastic, and interesting. They're also usually full of energy, spontaneous, and caring towards others, making them fun friends to be around. Plus, they can talk about many topics and have a wide range of interests, making them great conversationalists.

And even though impulsivity might seem like a bad thing, it can offer some unique benefits. It can make you more open to new experiences, which means you're open to trying new things and exploring new places. All these awesome qualities can make your social life more fulfilling and make you an awesome friend to have around.

Social skills to master

Social skills are our toolbox of skills that we can use to talk, listen, and interact with people around us. These skills include:

- Being a good listener
- Knowing how to communicate both verbally and non-verbally
- Having good relationships with others
- Being assertive
- Knowing how to handle conflicts
- Being able to persuade others
- Knowing how to delegate tasks effectively

These different tools in our social toolbox help build better relationships and communicate effectively.

Social competence & ADHD

As I've mentioned earlier, children with ADHD can sometimes find it harder to develop their social skills, which can make things a bit tougher for them as they grow up. For example, they might struggle to pick up on social cues or find it harder to make friends due to being excluded or isolated from social opportunities. As they become adults, they might still find that they struggle in a few areas:

- **Knowledge and skills**. They might not understand things like social rules or how to recognize and understand their and others' emotions. They could also find it hard to communicate verbally or non-verbally with others.
- **Performance deficit**. They might find it tough to pick up on non-verbal cues or struggle to regulate

their own behavior, which could cause them to offend others accidentally. They might also find it hard to solve problems or see things from other people's perspectives. Sometimes they can be more prone to emotional outbursts as they find it hard to regulate their emotions and might struggle to be aware of how they're doing socially.

Social rules

Have you ever felt like you've accidentally crossed a line with someone when you were chatting with them? Maybe you said something that was a bit too personal, or you invaded their personal space without realizing it. Well, it turns out that there are all these unspoken social rules that we're supposed to follow, and when we break them, it can make other people see us in a negative light. For example, there's a social rule that's all about respecting other people's boundaries. Everyone has their own ideas about what's okay and what's not when it comes to personal space, topics of conversation, and how much personal information they want to share with others. And if you're not careful, you could offend someone without even meaning to.

Some people might be ok with talking about religion or politics, while others would rather steer clear of those topics altogether. And then there are emotional outbursts or public displays of affection that some people might be fine with, while others might be uncomfortable with it. Basically, it's all about understanding what different people's boundaries are and making sure you respect them. It's not always easy, but it's vital to being a good friend, colleague, or just a decent human being.

Improving social competence

To become more socially competent, you can:

- Try to understand the unspoken social rules and concepts behind social thinking. That way, you'll better understand what's expected in different situations and what might be considered inappropriate.
- Work on your executive function skills. This might involve using medication to help regulate your thoughts, words, and behavior or coming up with other strategies to help you stay on track when you're interacting with others.
- Practice! It's the best way to get better at socializing. You can try consciously picking up on social clues, listening with both your ears and your eyes, taking other people's perspectives, and maintaining boundaries in conversation. It's all about being aware of your own behavior and being mindful of how others are reacting to you.

If you find yourself feeling overwhelmed or unsure of where to start, don't be afraid to reach out for help. A psychologist or an ADHD coach can provide guidance and support to help you improve your social competence.

Ways to master social skills

- **Knowledge** - Understanding what areas you need to work on can help improve your social skills. Read some relevant books, like "What Does Everybody Know That I Don't," to get some knowledge on the subject.
- **Attitude** - Keep a positive attitude and be open-minded about improving your social skills. Don't forget to appreciate feedback from others too! Accept compliments with grace, even if you're not on board with it.
- **Goals** - If you're an adult with ADHD, it might help focus on one goal at a time when working on your social skills. That way, you can really master each skill before moving on to the next one. You can start by assessing yourself and getting feedback from others to figure out what you need to work on.
- **The echo** - If you're someone who sometimes misses important information during conversations due to attention difficulties, try developing a system where you check in with the other person to make sure you understand them correctly. You could say something like, "I heard you say XYZ, did I get it right? Is there more?" And if you're the one providing important information, you could ask the other person to

repeat back what they heard you say. This can help prevent social errors that might happen because of inattention.

- **Observe others** - You can learn quite a bit by simply watching others do what you need to learn how to do. It might help choose some good role models both at work and in your personal life to help you improve in this area. And don't forget that TV can also be a great source of role models.
- **Role play** - One effective way for people with ADHD to enhance their social skills is by practicing the skills they need with other people. This can provide valuable feedback for improvement.
- **Visualization** - To improve their social skills, visualization can be a helpful tool. First decide which skill you want to work on and then rehearse it in your mind, imagining how you would apply it in different settings with specific people you'll be interacting with. By repeating this exercise, you can gain experience, which can increase your chances of success in real-world situations.
- **Prompts** - Using prompts can help stay on track with your social skill goals. Prompts can take various forms, such as a visual cue like an index card, a verbal reminder from someone, a physical cue like a vibrating watch set at intervals, or a simple gesture like someone scratching their head to remind you to work on your social skills.

- **Increase likeability** - Social exchange theory suggests that people stay in relationships based on how well those relationships meet their needs. Although people are not exactly "social accountants," they do evaluate the costs and benefits of being in relationships. People with ADHD are often considered to be "high maintenance," so it's important for you to consider what you can bring to relationships to balance things out. Research has identified several characteristics of highly likable people, including sincerity, honesty, understanding, loyalty, intelligence, thoughtfulness, and kindness. By working on developing or improving these characteristics, you can improve your social standing and strengthen your relationships.

Having ADHD can pose difficulties in maintaining social relationships, but there are resources available to help adults improve their social skills. Seeking help through reading, counseling, or coaching can be beneficial, but it's also important to build and maintain social connections.

ADHD AND RELATIONSHIPS

Dealing with ADHD in adult relationships can be tough, but it's not impossible. It's important to have compassion and work together as a team. Relationships require effort from both partners, and having ADHD can bring unique challenges to the table. Some partners may feel that individuals with ADHD are poor listeners, insensitive, easily distracted, or forgetful. These difficulties can strain even the most loving relationships. However, being aware of the impact of adult ADHD on relationships can help prevent breakups. With the right approach, it's possible to have a happy, fulfilling relationship despite the challenges.

Understanding ADHD

If you have a partner with ADHD, you may notice that they tend to be inattentive and hyperactive. We have discussed many of these difficulties at great length. You may find that your partner with ADHD has inappropriate outbursts which can be traumatizing to you and others. While these bursts of anger pass quickly, hurtful words spoken in the heat of the moment can be damaging.

ADHD and relationship difficulties

Although all individuals bring their own emotional baggage into a relationship, those with ADHD often struggle with specific challenges such as negative self-image, low self-esteem, and feelings of shame. Despite this, their ability to hyperfocus, a common ADHD symptom, allows them to shower their partner with affection and attention at the beginning of the relationship.

However, this hyperfocus is not sustainable, and when it shifts, the partner with ADHD may appear uninterested in their significant other. This can lead the neglected partner to question their partner's affection, creating strain in the relationship. Furthermore, the partner with ADHD may constantly doubt their significant other's love and commitment, which can be perceived as a lack of trust, leading to further disconnection between the couple.

ADHD and marriage

ADHD can significantly strain a marriage, with the non-ADHD spouse often taking on most responsibilities such as parenting, financial management, household chores, resolving family problems, and home management. This can create an imbalance in the relationship and make the partner with ADHD feel more like a child than an equal partner. This dynamic can lead to a loss of sexual intimacy and a feeling of disconnection, ultimately leading to divorce.

To cope with these challenges, it's important for both partners to practice empathy and focus on the reasons they fell in love. Small reminders of affection and appreciation can help carry the relationship through chaotic times. Yet if the strain becomes too much, it may be necessary to seek marriage counseling or couples therapy to address the issues and find solutions that work for both partners.

Why breakups happen

The partner with ADHD may sometimes be taken by surprise when a relationship ends, as they may have been too preoccupied to recognize that the relationship was deteriorating. To cope with the demands of daily life, the partner with ADHD may withdraw mentally and emotionally, leaving their partner feeling abandoned and resentful. If the partner with ADHD is undiagnosed or not receiving treatment, this dynamic can be exacerbated. Even with treatment, anger, and resentment may persist. Delaying the resolution of relationship problems can increase the likelihood of a breakup.

COMMUNICATION PROBLEMS

Every couple experiences conflicts as a natural part of their relationship. Yet not all couples possess the skills to effectively navigate these disagreements and move on, and those who do have a distinct advantage with a higher likelihood of achieving lasting happiness. For couples, including those with ADHD, the goal is not to avoid fighting altogether since it's inevitable, but to develop the ability to have constructive arguments or "good fights."

What science says

It's not about how often you argue that decides whether your relationship will last. It's more about how you deal with conflict and communicate to repair any damage that predicts the stability of a marriage. But here's the thing - ADHD relationships are more likely to have problems than others. Why, you ask? Partners with ADHD often have intense emotional reactions at the most unexpected moments. This can leave their partner, whether they have ADHD or not, feeling like they're walking on eggshells. Even worse, non-ADHD partners often fall into the habit of criticizing their spouse with ADHD, thinking they're helping by pushing them to be more organized and attentive. But this constant criticism just makes things worse. The person with ADHD feels like they're being verbally attacked and belittled, which leads to defensiveness and anger.

Communication tips

I want to share some ideas for fighting fairly and removing anger from fights.

- Don't criticize your partner
- Begin with a soft start or ease into the topic
- Always show respect to your partner
- Use non-threatening words and don't bully your partner
- Use clarifying phrases to ensure you both understand each other
- Try to remain calm and use mindfulness techniques to manage emotions
- Use pre-agreed verbal cues to take a break from the conversation
- Make eye contact to show that you are engaged
- Look for common ground to solve the problem together
- Ask open-ended questions and listen to your partner's response

- Use affirming statements to show you hear your partner's concern
- Accept the legitimacy of negative emotions and commiserate with your partner

MORE RELATIONSHIP TIPS: WAYS TO SAVE YOUR RELATIONSHIP

Falling in love is a natural feeling, even for adults with ADHD. The rush of chemicals in your brain during the initial phase of love is not unique. However, it's easy to hyperfocus on romantic feelings to increase the dopamine levels that are often lacking in our brains. But intense emotions alone cannot sustain a lasting relationship. It takes more than that to make an ADHD relationship work. Let's face it, relationships are hard. We can't just rely on love to make them work. We need practical coping skills to overcome our weaknesses and keep the relationship going. So, what kind of tools should you have in your relationship toolbox if your partner has ADHD? Great question.

Manage symptoms

Take responsibility for managing adult ADHD by using behavior therapy or appropriate medication to manage symptoms, increase dopamine levels, and improve brain function. By doing so, you can expect a reduction in ADHD symptoms like struggling to focus when your partner speaks or completing tasks like paying bills on time.

One common issue in relationships with ADHD partners is the feeling of not being heard. To improve your listening skills, try giving your partner five minutes to talk while maintaining eye contact and leaning in. Summarize what you heard, then you can then do something you enjoy. This exercise will likely surprise your partner and make them feel heard.

Commit to commitment

ADHD can affect relationships in both positive and negative ways due to symptoms like impulsiveness and a need for constant stimulation. This can make it challenging to maintain monogamy and prioritize the idea of a relationship. It's essential to stay committed to the institution of a relationship, even more than to your partner.

Use laughter therapy

It can help find humor in your ADHD symptoms rather than getting upset by them. Rather than taking unintended words and actions personally, recognize them as symptoms of your condition. Laughing about it can help you move forward in your relationship. It's understandable to feel defensive about ADHD symptoms, but letting go of that defensiveness can be beneficial.

Forgive and forget

Blaming the other person for problems in the relationship is a common trap, but it takes two people to make things work.

By admitting to the problems you may be causing rather than focusing on your partner's mistakes, you can grow emotionally. When you acknowledge our own weaknesses, work on them. It becomes easier to accept your partner and forgive their shortcomings. A phrase that encapsulates this idea of forgiveness is, "I did my best in that moment. If I could have done better, I would have." This helps to remove the hurt from a negative experience and allows you and your partner to have civil conversations. It's no longer about someone "doing it again," but about being human and making mistakes, which is something that can be forgiven.

Seek professional help

Couples with ADHD often plan to stay together forever, but unresolved issues can grow into insurmountable problems. Don't wait until it's too late to seek professional help. A licensed therapist can teach communication and conflict resolution skills to prevent divorce.

FINDING THE RIGHT ONE

Having ADHD can make social relationships tricky. It can be tough to pay attention to others, keep up with cues, and control mood swings or impulses. Finding the right partner can help, but it's important to address negative patterns too. Dating or getting back into it can be exciting, but also nerve-wracking. How do you know if they're a good match? How do you handle the risk of heartbreak?

Make a list

Start by making a list of what you want in a partner. Think about what qualities are important to you, like excitement, stability, or shared values and interests. Also consider your relationship goals; are you looking for something fun and casual or a serious, long-term commitment? If you're currently seeing someone, make a list of their good qualities, what you're attracted to, and any concerns you may have. If they have ADHD, are they taking steps to manage it? How do you feel around them? Are you comfortable being yourself? And most importantly, is this someone you can see yourself with for the long haul?

Enlist a trusted friend

Sometimes it's good to chat with a close friend or family member who supports you to help you make sense of things. When you're in the middle of a new relationship, it's easy to get carried away and lose your objectivity. Plus, you might miss some important red flags that someone on the outside could spot for you.

Review your relationship history

Take some time to reflect on your past relationships and identify any patterns that may be present. Have you noticed that you tend to jump into relationships headfirst, only to lose interest after the initial excitement wears off? Have you found yourself attracted to the wrong type of person because you miss important social cues? Do you struggle to connect with your partner on an intimate level, or do your impulsive reactions cause problems in the relationship? Are you prone to picking fights or sabotaging the relationship in some way? And have you stayed in a bad relationship for too long, hoping that the other person would change? Being honest with yourself about these patterns can help you break free from them and create healthier relationships in the future.

Develop positive strategies

Once you've recognized previous relationship challenges, focus on finding solutions. For those with ADHD, the most challenging areas often relate to self-control deficits like distractibility and inattention that can be interpreted by a partner as indifference, problems managing emotions, and impulses that can cause hurt feelings.

Taking medication can often help reduce the intensity of these symptoms. Techniques like positive self-talk, role-playing, practicing good communication, becoming more conscious of emotional triggers, and taking time to relax can all help in developing and maintaining healthy relationships.

Practice honest communication

To have a healthy relationship, communication is key. Start by being friends and regularly assess how the relationship is progressing. If there are any issues, approach them constructively and without blame. Focus on solutions, not problems. If you tend to talk a lot, try to listen more. Show interest in your partner and plan enjoyable activities together. Build trust and respect over time by taking it slow, laughing together, and being honest with each other.

SUMMARY

- With education and proper treatment, people with ADHD can learn strategies to improve social skills and form positive relationships
- Some ADHD symptoms, such as curiosity can make you more open to new experiences
- You can practice and improve your social skills through various strategies
- To manage relationships when you have ADHD, commit to the commitment you made, use laughter therapy, forgive and forget, and seek professional help
- As a person with ADHD, you can find the right person who will appreciate and love you

Cultivating healthy relationships and developing social skills is essential for individuals to lead fulfilling lives. By identifying past relationship problems, working on solutions, and practicing effective communication and active listening, individuals can build and maintain healthy relationships. Developing social skills through social activities and therapy can also help individuals improve their interactions with others and lead to better emotional and mental health. With effort and dedication, anyone can improve their social skills and build strong, supportive relationships.

It is clear to see that we have come a long way in understanding ADHD, but there is still a way to go still. Ultimately ADHD is not so bad, and with the right tools and strategies, alongside medication, anyone with ADHD can live a full and wonderful life.

CONCLUSION

Understanding ADHD, especially in women, is a huge step towards breaking down the stigma and misconceptions that surround it. You should never feel ashamed or flawed for having ADHD as a woman. With the right tools and understanding, women with ADHD can have fulfilling and successful lives, personally and professionally. Just look at some of the amazing famous women with ADHD who are making a difference in their fields!

In relationships, communication is key. Learning to manage emotions and developing healthy social skills can make a huge difference in cultivating healthy and positive relationships. With practice and patience, women with ADHD can build strong connections and meaningful partnerships. And who doesn't love a heartwarming love story?!

In the workplace, women with ADHD can excel in their careers by finding their strengths and building on them. The key is to develop effective strategies to manage time, prioritize tasks, and stay focused. With the right support and accommodations, women with ADHD can thrive in their careers and achieve their goals.

Managing emotions is another crucial aspect of living with ADHD. By recognizing and understanding their emotions, women with ADHD can develop effective coping strategies and lead happier, healthier lives.

Finally, the importance of healthy eating cannot be overstated. A balanced diet can have a significant impact on managing symptoms of ADHD and improving overall health and well-being.

So, to all the women with ADHD out there: embrace who you are, find your strengths, and don't let anyone tell you that you can't achieve your dreams. With the right tools and support, the sky is the limit!

COMING SOON!

Attention all ADHD warriors and relationship seekers!

Are you tired of feeling like your ADHD is getting in the way of your relationships? Are you ready to take your connections to the next level and build the kind of fulfilling relationships you deserve and desire? Then get excited and ready for the relationship revolution with my upcoming book on how to build meaningful relationships when you have ADHD.

In this groundbreaking book, I draw on years of research, personal experience, and insights from experts in the field to provide you with a comprehensive guide to navigating relationships when you have ADHD. Packed with **practical advice, real-world solutions, and empowering insights**, this book is your ticket to overcoming the challenges of ADHD and thriving in your relationships like never before.

Whether you're struggling to maintain personal or professional relationships, dealing with the fallout of impulsive behavior, or simply looking for ways to improve your overall relationship satisfaction, I've got you covered. With a focus on real-world solutions and strategies, this book will give you the tools you need to overcome the challenges of ADHD and build healthy and lasting relationships.

So don't wait – sign up for updates at **RoSirisena@Young-womenwithadhd.com** and be the first to know when this game-changing book hits the shelves. With its powerful message and transformative advice, a must-read for anyone looking to build stronger, healthier connections in their life. Get ready to take your relationships to the next level!

Feel free to connect with me at **RoSirisena@Youngwomen-withadhd.com**

REFERENCES

Additude. (2011, October 11). *ADHD Awareness Week: ADD Statistics About Anxiety, Sleep, Work*. ADDitude. Retrieved March 23, 2023, from https://www.additudemag.com/staggering-new-statistics-about-adhd/

Additude. (2022, June 24). *Benefits of ADHD / ADD: Love Your Strengths and Abilities*. ADDitude. Retrieved March 9, 2023, from https://www.additudemag.com/slideshows/benefits-of-adhd-to-love/

Additude. (2023, February 8). *ADHD Diet Plan: Foods to Eat & Avoid to Help ADD Symptoms*. ADDitude. Retrieved March 12, 2023, from https://www.additudemag.com/adhd-diet-nutrition-sugar/

ADHD and Women. (2021, October 16). *Today, I am a doctor! – ADHD and Women*. ADHD and Women. Retrieved March 9, 2023, from https://adhd-women.eu/blog/today-i-am-a-doctor/

Attention Deficit Disorder Association (ADDA). (n.d.). *Should I Disclose My ADHD? | ADHD At Work*. ADHD At Work. Retrieved March 23, 2023, from https://adhdatwork.add.org/disclosing-adhd-at-work/

Barrow, K. (2022, March 31). *Famous Women with ADHD Who Learned to Shine*. ADDitude. Retrieved March 9, 2023, from https://www.additudemag.com/famous-women-with-adhd-work/

Batten, L. (2022, August 17). *How ADHD Is Different in Women – Frida*. Frida. Retrieved March 2, 2023, from https://www.talkwithfrida.com/learn/how-is-adhd-different-in-women/#how-symptoms-of-adhd-differ-in-women

Beauchaine, T. P., Ben-David, I., & Bos, M. (2020). ADHD, financial distress, and suicide in adulthood: A population study. *Science Advances, 6*, 40. https://doi.org/10.1126/sciadv.aba1551

Bonvissuto, D. (2018, January 8). *Should I Tell My Boss I Have ADHD?* WebMD. Retrieved March 23, 2023, from https://www.webmd.com/add-adhd/features/boss-adhd

Brown, T. E. (2022, June 20). *How ADHD Triggers Intense Emotions In Your Brain*. ADDitude. Retrieved March 16, 2023, from https://www.addi

tudemag.com/slideshows/adhd-emotions-understanding-intense-feelings/

Caldwell, M. (n.d.). *The Power of Gratitude — ADDept.* ADDept. Retrieved March 19, 2023, from https://www.addept.org/living-with-adult-add-adhd/the-power-of-gratitude

Cassata, C., & Young, A. (2023, February 13). *What Is Norepinephrine? How It Affects the Body and How It's Used in Medication.* Everyday Health. Retrieved March 2, 2023, from https://www.everydayhealth.com/norepinephrine/guide/

Centers For Disease Control And Prevention (CDC). (n.d.). *Symptoms and Diagnosis of ADHD | CDC.* Centers for Disease Control and Prevention. Retrieved March 2, 2023, from https://www.cdc.gov/ncbddd/adhd/diagnosis.html

Children and Adults with Attention-Deficit/Hyperactivity Disorder (CHADD). (n.d.). *Managing Money and ADHD: Expenses and Goals.* CHADD. Retrieved March 21, 2023, from https://chadd.org/for-adults/managing-money-and-adhd-expenses-and-goals/

Children and Adults with Attention-Deficit/Hyperactivity Disorder (CHADD). (n.d.). *Managing Money and ADHD: Minding Your Debts.* CHADD. Retrieved March 21, 2023, from https://chadd.org/for-adults/managing-money-and-adhd-minding-your-debts/

Children and Adults with Attention-Deficit/Hyperactivity Disorder (CHADD). (n.d.). *Managing Money and ADHD: Money Management Schedule.* CHADD. Retrieved March 21, 2023, from https://chadd.org/for-adults/managing-money-and-adhd-money-management-schedule/

Children and Adults with Attention-Deficit/Hyperactivity Disorder (CHADD). (n.d.). *Managing Money and ADHD: Saving and Spending.* CHADD. Retrieved March 21, 2023, from https://chadd.org/for-adults/managing-money-and-adhd-saving-and-spending/

Children and Adults with Attention-Deficit/Hyperactivity Disorder (CHADD). (n.d.). *Myths and Misunderstandings.* CHADD. Retrieved March 2, 2023, from https://chadd.org/about-adhd/myths-and-misunderstandings/

Children and Adults with Attention-Deficit/Hyperactivity Disorder (CHADD). (n.d.). *Relationships & Social Skills.* CHADD. Retrieved March 23, 2023, from https://chadd.org/for-adults/relationships-social-skills/

Children and Adults with Attention-Deficit/Hyperactivity Disorder (CHADD). (2019, April 4). *Rejection Can Be More Painful with ADHD.* CHADD. Retrieved March 17, 2023, from https://chadd.org/adhd-weekly/rejection-can-more-painful-with-adhd/

Children and Adults with Attention-Deficit/Hyperactivity Disorder (CHADD). (2019, October 17). *Managing Stress When You Have ADHD.* CHADD. Retrieved March 15, 2023, from https://chadd.org/adhd-weekly/managing-stress-when-you-have-adhd/

Cooper, J., & Nadeau, K. (n.d.). *Your Lifestyle Will Determine Your Future.* CHADD. Retrieved March 11, 2023, from https://chadd.org/adhd-news/adhd-news-adults/your-lifestyle-will-determine-your-future/

Dickson, M. (n.d.). *Melissa's ADHD love story: impulsive first dates, beating cancer and a happy ending.* Kaleidoscope Society. Retrieved March 23, 2023, from https://www.kaleidoscopesociety.com/adhd-love-story-impulsive-first-dates-beating-cancer-and-a-happy-ending/

Ditzell, J. (2022, May 18). *ADHD and Emotions: Relationship and Tips to Manage.* Healthline. Retrieved March 16, 2023, from https://www.healthline.com/health/adhd/emotional-regulation#adhd-and-emotions

Dodson, W. (2023, January 20). *How ADHD Ignites Rejection Sensitive Dysphoria.* ADDitude. Retrieved March 17, 2023, from https://www.additudemag.com/rejection-sensitive-dysphoria-and-adhd/

Flippin, R. (2021, January 25). *ADHD at Work: Time Wasters and Productivity Killers.* ADDitude. Retrieved March 23, 2023, from https://www.additudemag.com/adhd-at-work-time-wasters-and-productivity-killers/

Footprints To Recovery. (n.d.). *7 Ways to Combat Negative Self-Talk.* Footprints to Recovery. Retrieved March 10, 2023, from https://footprintstorecovery.com/blog/combat-negative-self-talk/

Gepp, K. (2022, May 2). *ADHD and Self-Esteem: What's the Connection?* Healthline. Retrieved March 9, 2023, from https://www.healthline.com/health/adhd/adhd-and-self-esteem#when-to-reach-out

Gil, N. (2022, October 23). *How ADHD Makes Money More Complicated For Women.* Refinery29. Retrieved March 20, 2023, from https://www.refinery29.com/en-gb/adhd-costing-women-money

Hall, J. (2022, December 16). *18 Time Management Tips for People with ADHD.* Calendar App. Retrieved March 23, 2023, from https://www.calendar.com/blog/18-time-management-tips-for-people-with-adhd/

Halverstadt, J. (2021, January 21). *ADHD and Relationships: 10 Rules for Adults with ADHD / ADD*. ADDitude. Retrieved March 23, 2023, from https://www.additudemag.com/save-your-adhd-relationship-marriage/

Hassall, J. (2020, October). *Adult ADHD and Emotions*. CHADD. Retrieved March 16, 2023, from https://chadd.org/attention-article/adult-adhd-and-emotions/

Ivey, A. G. (2022, July 11). *Common Workplace ADHD Problems and How to Fix Them*. WebMD. Retrieved March 23, 2023, from https://www.webmd.com/add-adhd/common-adhd-workplace-problems

Jaksa, P. (2022, July 1). *How to Regain Your Confidence: Life-Changing Strategies for Adults with ADHD*. ADDitude. Retrieved March 10, 2023, from https://www.additudemag.com/how-to-regain-self-confidence-adults-adhd/

Juby, B. (2022, July 20). *Understanding the Connection Between ADHD and Messiness*. Healthline. Retrieved March 22, 2023, from https://www.healthline.com/health/adhd-and-messy#tips-for-getting-organized

Kolberg, J. (2022, July 13). *How to Get Organized with Adult ADHD: Organization with ADD*. ADDitude. Retrieved March 22, 2023, from https://www.additudemag.com/how-to-get-organized-with-adhd/

Kubala, K. (2022, April 12). *ADHD and Social Skills: What to Know*. Psych Central. Retrieved March 23, 2023, from https://psychcentral.com/adhd/adhd-social-skills#benefits

Lener, M. S., & Cronkleton, E. (2021, August 12). *ADHD brain vs. normal brain: Function, differences, and more*. Medical News Today. Retrieved March 2, 2023, from https://www.medicalnewstoday.com/articles/adhd-brain-vs-normal-brain#structure

Levine, H. (2022, January 17). *How Mindful Meditation and Yoga Can Help Treat ADHD*. WebMD. Retrieved March 21, 2023, from https://www.webmd.com/add-adhd/adhd-mindfulness-meditation-yoga

Low, K. (2020, September 18). *Finding the Right Dating Partner When You Have ADHD*. Verywell Mind. Retrieved March 23, 2023, from https://www.verywellmind.com/dating-and-add-20384

Low, K. (2020, December 21). *How to Avoid Impulsive Spending With ADHD*. Verywell Mind. Retrieved March 21, 2023, from https://www.verywellmind.com/is-impulsive-spending-breaking-your-budget-20378

Matthews, J. (2022, July 8). *ADHD Symptoms in Women That Doctors Miss or*

Don't Believe. ADDitude. Retrieved March 16, 2023, from https://www.additudemag.com/adhd-symptoms-in-women-stories/

Maynard, S. (2022, March 11). *Making Peace With Your Clutter: A Guide for ADHD Adults*. ADDitude. Retrieved March 22, 2023, from https://www.additudemag.com/making-peace-with-your-clutter/

Meijer, S. (2019, May 30). *ADHD can make it harder to manage your money. Here's some tips to help*. ABC. Retrieved March 20, 2023, from https://www.abc.net.au/news/2019-05-31/how-adhd-affects-your-wallet-mental-health-kids/11158952

Minnis, G. (2021, October 19). *ADHD and Exercise: What You Need to Know*. Healthline. Retrieved March 14, 2023, from https://www.healthline.com/health/fitness/adhd-and-exercise#exercises-for-adults-with-adhd

Morein-Zamir, S., Kasese, M., Chamberlain, S., & Trachtenberg, E. (2021, December 13). *Elevated levels of hoarding in ADHD: a special link with inattention*. NCBI. Retrieved March 21, 2023, from https://www.ncbi.nlm.nih.gov/pmc/articles/PMC7612156/

National Health Service (NHS). (n.d.). *Attention deficit hyperactivity disorder (ADHD) - Causes*. NHS. Retrieved March 2, 2023, from https://www.nhs.uk/conditions/attention-deficit-hyperactivity-disorder-adhd/causes/

National Health Service (NHS). (n.d.). *Attention deficit hyperactivity disorder (ADHD) - Symptoms*. NHS. Retrieved March 2, 2023, from https://www.nhs.uk/conditions/attention-deficit-hyperactivity-disorder-adhd/symptoms/

National Health Service (NHS). (n.d.). *Overview - - - Attention deficit hyperactivity disorder (ADHD)*. NHS. Retrieved March 2, 2023, from https://www.nhs.uk/conditions/attention-deficit-hyperactivity-disorder-adhd/

Olivardia, R. (2022, March 31). *Healthy Eating Habits for Adults with ADHD*. ADDitude. Retrieved March 12, 2023, from https://www.additudemag.com/healthy-eating-habits-adhd-adults/

Orlov, M. (2021, May 20). *ADHD and Marriage: Communication Problems and Fixes*. ADDitude. Retrieved March 23, 2023, from https://www.additudemag.com/marriage-communication-adhd-spouses/

Pacheco, D. (2023, February 9). *ADHD and Sleep Problems: How Are They Related?* Sleep Foundation. Retrieved March 12, 2023, from https://www.sleepfoundation.org/mental-health/adhd-and-sleep

Safai, Y. (2023, March 8). *How ADHD Affects Relationships And What You Can*

Do. Healthline. Retrieved March 23, 2023, from https://www.healthline.com/health/adhd/adult-adhd-relationships#adhd-and-marriage

Segal, R., & Smith, M. (2022, December 30). *Treatment for Adult ADHD*. HelpGuide.org. Retrieved March 2, 2023, from https://www.helpguide.org/articles/add-adhd/treatment-for-adult-adhd-attention-deficit-disorder.htm

Sherman, C. (2023, February 8). *Mindful Meditation for ADHD: Natural Remedy for ADD Symptoms*. ADDitude. Retrieved March 21, 2023, from https://www.additudemag.com/mindfulness-meditation-for-adhd/

Silver, L. (2023, January 21). *The ADHD Brain: Neuroscience Behind Attention Deficit Disorder*. ADDitude. Retrieved March 2, 2023, from https://www.additudemag.com/neuroscience-of-adhd-brain/

Smith, J. (2021, June 29). *ADHD and Empathy: Identifying and Resolving the Disconnect*. FastBraiin. Retrieved March 18, 2023, from https://www.fastbraiin.com/blogs/blog/adhd-and-empathy

Steed, L. (2022, October 25). *How to Show Empathy: Advice for ADHD Brains*. ADDitude. Retrieved March 17, 2023, from https://www.additudemag.com/how-to-show-empathy-adhd-friendship/

Strong, R. (2022, September 11). *Can ADHD Affect Empathy? It's Complicated*. Mindpath Health. Retrieved March 18, 2023, from https://www.mindpath.com/resource/can-adhd-affect-empathy-its-complicated/

Thriving With ADHD. (n.d.). *Developing Social Competence*. Thriving with ADHD. Retrieved March 23, 2023, from https://thrivingwithadhd.com.au/developing-social-competence/

Tuckman, A. (2022, August 12). *Time Management Skills for ADHD Brains: Practical Advice*. ADDitude. Retrieved March 23, 2023, from https://www.additudemag.com/time-management-skills-adhd-brain/

Watson, S. (2022, August 25). *Adult ADHD at Work: Tips for Organization and Control*. WebMD. Retrieved March 23, 2023, from https://www.webmd.com/add-adhd/adhd-in-the-workplace

Woodruff, L. (2022, February 10). *How to Organize Your Home When You Have ADHD*. ADDitude. Retrieved March 22, 2023, from https://www.additudemag.com/home-organization-with-adhd/

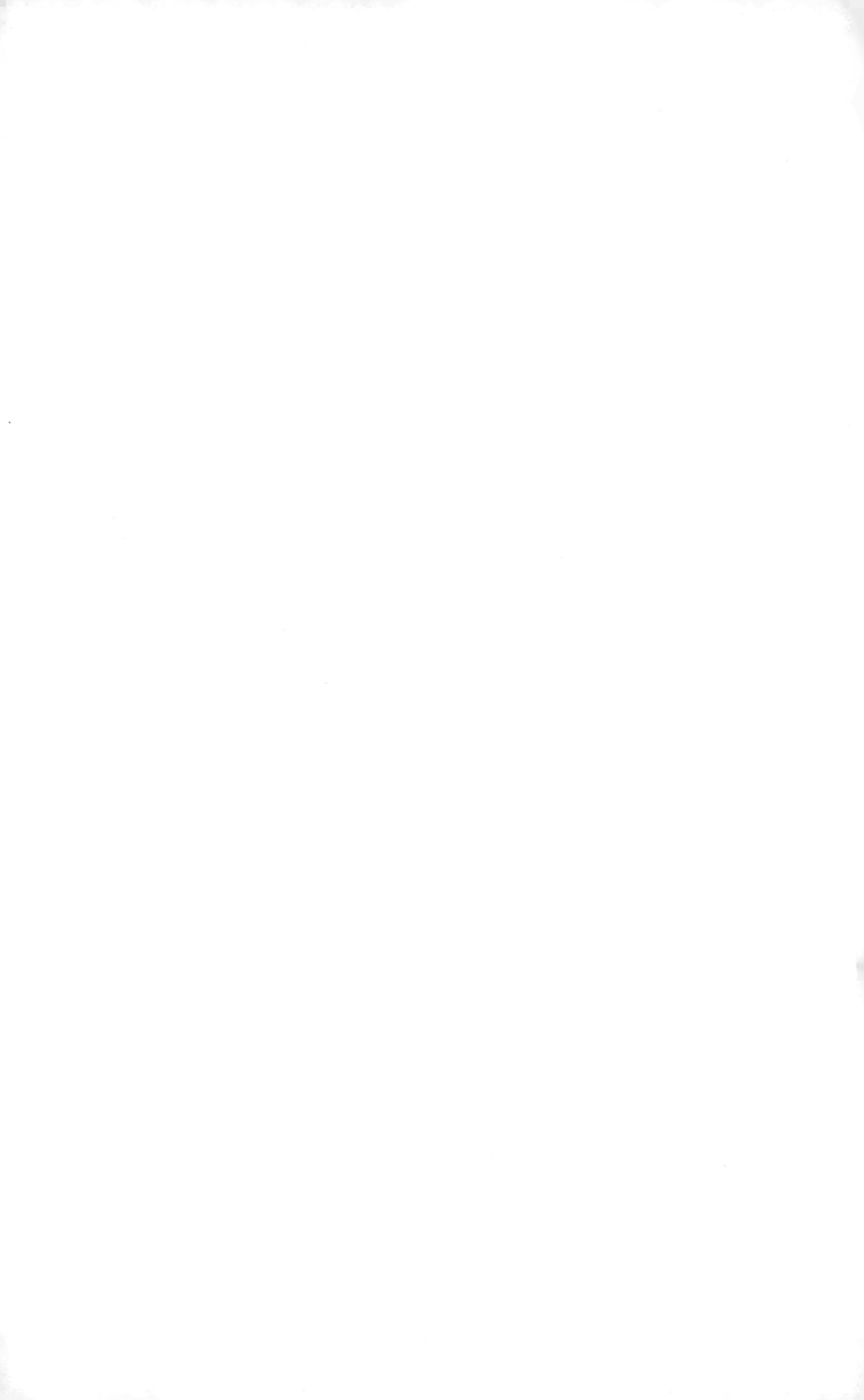